SALT
KILLS

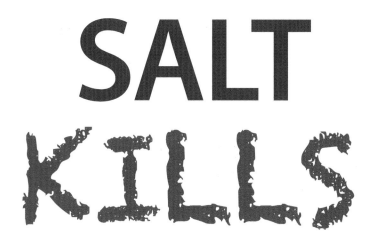

SALT KILLS

Surender Reddy Neravetla, MD, FACS
Director
Cardiac Surgery
Springfield Regional Medical Center

with
Shantanu Reddy Neravetla, MD
Transitional Intern
Virginia Mason Medical Center

Health Now Books, LLC
Springfield, Ohio

Health Now Books, LLC
3484 Rockview Drive
Springfield, Ohio 45504
healthnowbooks.com

ISBN: 978-1-938009-00-6   (full-color book)

ISBN: 978-1-938009-01-3   (black and white book)

ISBN: 978-1-938009-02-0   (ePub e-book)

Library of Congress Control Number: 2012900551

For more information
about salt and other health-related issues,
please visit healthnowbooks.com.

Acknowledgments

My first thanks go to my immediate family members, who not only helped with the actual work, they put up with me during the entire project.

Thanks also go to my extended family, including my office workers, my assistants, the surgery team and the many colleagues who participated in the thought process and provided a sounding board.

Thanks to Tina Pavlatos from Visual Anatomy for producing excellent illustrations and putting my ideas into pictures, as well as to Jennifer Omner for the book's design and layout.

Finally, thanks to my writing coach and editor Linden Gross, who helped me formulate my ideas and make my case as clearly and strongly as I possibly could.

Contents

Preface

"Please take good care of him," pleads the 50-year-old mother of three children, as we are getting ready to take her husband to the operating room. She holds my hand firmly with both her hands and continues tearfully, "We have been married for 30 years and I don't want to lose him now." The rest of the family is huddled on the other side of the bed holding each other. The anxiety and worry is very clear in their eyes. I reassure her one last time, and finally she lets go of my hand. The surgery team then takes him into the operating room.

The patient and the family have placed the life of their loved one in the hands of my team and have complete faith in us. We take this responsibility very seriously. Once we decide to perform open-heart surgery on a patient, we have many conversations with the patient and family members. The members of my team and I go over the options for treatment, what to expect from the operation, and walk them through all the steps leading up to the surgery. A certain bond invariably develops between us. We are a community-based hospital in the Midwest, the heartland of America, where this type of scene occurs day in and day out.

The surgery goes well. Coronary artery bypass surgery, the most common heart surgery performed, builds new pathways for the blood supply to the heart muscle, to make up for the arteries blocked by fat buildup. We constructed bypasses for three arteries on this patient's heart. More than a quarter million of these surgeries are performed every year in the United States.

Now that the surgery is finished, it is time again to talk to the family. The gathering has gotten even bigger. The neighbors, the pastor, friends, and siblings are all anxiously waiting. I inform the gathering that the patient has an enlarged heart, there is some damage to the heart muscle from previous heart attacks and there are multiple blocked arteries. All of this is a common finding. Three bypasses were done! We expect a normal recovery barring any unusual problems. Everybody breathes a sigh of relief. The overweight son with cigarettes hanging out of his pocket exclaims, "The problem is solved; he's as good as new!"

No, the problem has been solved only temporarily. We just bypassed the existing blockages. The blockages will continue to build unless the patient changes what created the blockages in the first place.

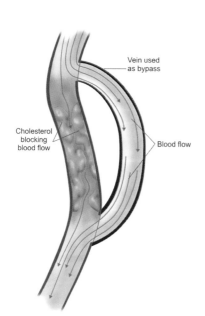

Vein used as bypass

Cholesterol blocking blood flow

Blood flow

Cholesterol, once built into the arteries, cannot be removed except in a few locations. What we do is build a detour around the blocked artery, hence "bypass surgery." The enlarged heart is not likely to get better, either. If the heart continues to grow bigger, this alone can lead to heart failure.

These concepts confuse many in the family. "What do we need to do?" they ask. I give advice along the usual party lines: stop smoking, eat healthy and exercise regularly.

The wife protests, "Since the last heart attack he has done all that."

The last check-up showed that the cholesterol level had come down to a normal level with medications. So why did the cholesterol continue to build?

This is an all too frequent dilemma. The patient has gone through a life-changing experience and the entire crowd is concerned about what is next and who might be next in line for the same problem. They're looking for answers.

This is a critical point. I have physically handled and repaired their loved one's heart. No guesswork; this is as real as it gets. With a reprieve at hand, they are highly receptive and primed to receive good advice. I have a golden opportunity to make a serious impact on the health of this gathering. I feel a certain urge and sense of responsibly to find and give *real* advice. But what exactly do I tell them that will help?

Before the next surgery, I go into the physicians' lounge for some refreshment. Only physicians can enter here. The doughnuts have been devoured, but one cookie is left. The bags of chips are almost gone. Nobody has touched the apples or the oranges; as usual, they will probably rot away. Only the bananas have been eaten.

A soup and salad bar has recently been added to our lounge. One of my colleagues selects a salad and proceeds to drown it in a salty and fatty dressing. The other one opts for a bowl of salty soup and adds salty crackers to it. In turn, each of them picks up the saltshaker and adds even more salt to the salad and soup.

All this time, the local newspaper is opened on the table to the page with the recommendation from the Department of Health and Agriculture Forum to cut salt intake. Look what the physicians are doing with their own health! You would think they would be better informed and act accordingly.

Whenever any discussion of heart disease comes up, excess animal fat consumption usually gets the blame. But on a recent trip to India to visit my family, I got a big surprise. My relatives' typical daily food intake does not include any animal protein at all; they rarely eat meat of any kind. Yet just about everybody over the age of 50 that I knew had high blood pressure. Very high blood pressure indeed. Hardly any exceptions! The ones who thought they did *not* have it actually had untreated high blood pressure, which is even worse. Obviously, animal fat is not a major contributor to their poor health. Yet diabetes and heart problems are all rampant in spite of their predominantly vegetarian diets. All of them are gulping down multiple medications and supplements.

Do we all need to be on dozens of medications and supplements by the time we are nearing retirement age? Do we all need to go through expensive and painful procedures and surgeries? What are we doing to ourselves? Is there no way out? Who is next? Is this how we are going to spend our golden years?

All of these experiences led me to examine more closely the real root causes of cardiovascular health problems. Over the years—as a surgeon and as a concerned citizen—I have come across extensive published information. It is my passion to look at the health news regularly, not simply to read the headlines but to trace it to the source. In short, I have become a **health news junkie**. And that has helped me figure out the seeming health contradictions I've just described.

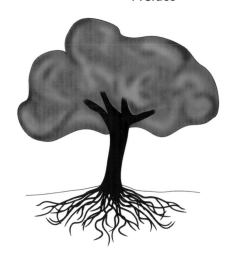

To me, it is as clear as day. The evidence is abundant. There are overlooked **root causes** of cardiovascular health problems. Many people inside and outside the medical community are not fully aware of—or not paying enough attention to—this information. Most people decide to practice good health habits only after a serious health problem has occurred. The majority of these problems actually have their beginnings in the early years of life. Once high blood pressure, diabetes, heart disease, etc., have developed, it is already too late. They cannot be cured. The best you can hope for is to keep them under control. We simply have to place a much stronger, higher priority on prevention than on treatment.

To make this point, let us look at the following illustration.

You wake up one morning to find the bathroom floor is flooded. You use a mop to clear the water off the floor. But a faucet has been left running though the night and the drain is plugged. Unless this faucet is turned off, the water on the floor can never be completely mopped up. The running faucet and plugged drain are the real root causes. What most people are doing is merely mopping. All the latest technology, newer medications, latest surgical techniques and procedures are noth-ing but fancier forms of the mop. They do not address the leaky faucet or the plugged drain.

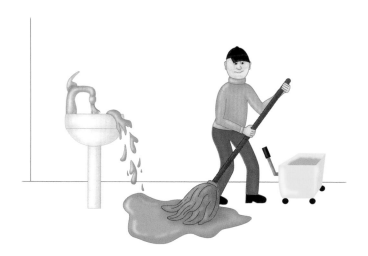

Looking at it another way:

The beautiful flower garden that is your life has started growing weeds. These weeds initially went unnoticed. Some of them now have their roots intertwined with the roots of flower-ing plants. At this stage, the root of the weed cannot be removed without damaging the flower-ing plant. Without eliminating the root, the weed will reap-pear. You may be able to keep it under control with repeated trimming but you have to accept living with the weed in your garden. It is an incurable ill.

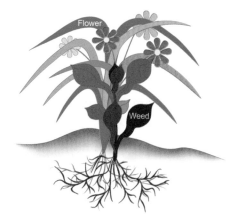

Many chronic illnesses are like these weeds; their roots are deeply intertwined with the flowering plant of life. Understanding of this simple analogy hopefully will get us to focus on the urgent need for better health habits—before the weeds begin to take over the garden.

During my years of research, I have come across very real root causes for many of our health problems. Adding salt to our food is one such root cause—or, if you will, one leaky faucet. We have grown accustomed to salting our food without realizing how dangerous the consequences are. The seed for this deadly weed has been planted and nurtured by us. We need to stop nurturing this weed. This salt faucet needs to be turned off.

This book, the first of a series of books dedicated to healthy living, focuses entirely on the problem of excess salt consumption. Let us start by learning the dangers of consuming excess salt.

1. Do you know the real root causes of your health problems?
2. Do you know that there are weeds growing in the garden of your health?
3. Are you just mopping the wet floor without turning the faucet off?
4. Are you content with taking a bowl of pills every day, going through expensive procedures and surgeries?
5. Are you content with the idea of living out your golden years in pain and with functional limitations?

Don't depend on the mop.

Unplug the drain.

Turn the faucet off.

Chapter

1

The Killer in Your Kitchen

"Salt kills? Really? Are you talking about the same salt that is in the shakers on every table in every restaurant across the world? The same salt added to every packaged food and most drinks that we buy? The same salt that we add to every preparation in our own kitchen and add some extra on the dining table? *That* salt? It *kills*?" I've heard reactions like this many, many times.

Salt kills! Yes, it does. There is no other way to put it except to put it bluntly, succinctly, straight up and firmly. And that is not all. This salt that you so routinely use causes extensive disability and dysfunction in many organ systems of the body, affecting many times more people than the number who have died from causes other than salt.

You know that smoking is bad news. For decades, smoking has been understood to be the number one cause of preventable death and disability. All the cancers that come from smoking, heart disease, emphysema, etc., are all well-known preventable health problems. Just don't smoke.

But scientists from prominent universities, with research sponsored by the World Health Organization, are now saying *our salt habit is the number one preventable health problem.* Isn't that shocking?

Let's get an overview of the extensive health problems that come from simply adding salt to our food and find out why salt is called Public Enemy Number One.

Salt: Public Enemy Number One

I woke up to see the headlines flashing everywhere. America had finally caught up with Osama bin Laden, the "most wanted" person ever. I remember 9/11 very vividly. In the middle of surgery, one of my assistants came running into the room shouting, "A big passenger plane hit one of the twin towers in New York!" I could not believe it. I barely finished the surgery and ran into the lounge where a big crowd was gathered. Everybody was glued to the TV. Right then another large passenger plane slammed into the second tower. The sight of the towers crumbling down and images of desperate people jumping to their deaths from the high floors disturbed me for a long time, even though I deal with death every day.

Close to 3,000 people perished in those buildings that day. Subsequently, during the invasion of Afghanistan, nearly 1,500 American soldiers lost their lives. The Iraq war death toll of American lives is currently estimated at 4,500. These events also changed the way we live—permanently. The amount of money and resources spent to defend ourselves has been astronomical. We still don't feel safe, do we?

Let us look at another calamity. On April 26, 2011, an earthquake triggered a massive tsunami in the northern islands of Japan. I happened to see an amateur video shot from a hilltop as the massive wave gushed through the town carrying all the houses, cars, roads, and bridges with it. People who were at the leading edge of the wave were running as hard as they could to get to higher ground. Just imagine the commotion. The death toll is approaching 15,000, with more unaccounted for. At least

100,000 people have been displaced. So many lives affected forever by a catastrophe over which they have no control. Understandably, the government of Japan is engaged in a massive relief effort.

Let us compare these and many similar events to the devastation caused by preventable health problems, specifically health problems that can be sidestepped simply by reducing salt in your diet. In my own extended family and in my neighborhood, there are any number of examples of diabetes, high blood pressure, heart disease, osteoporosis, asthma, stroke, stomach cancer and, of course, dementia. Pretty much every household is dealing with more than one of these issues. Is it just a problem with my family or my neighborhood? Not at all.

A brief look at each one of these health issues, which we'll explore in greater depth later on, will make the point that salt should be considered a bigger killer than 9/11 and the recent wars and calamities combined.

Most people know by now (or should know) that salt is responsible for high blood pressure and heart problems. But do you know that salt consumption contributes significantly to all these other problems?

For starters, dementia (loss of memory) is a worldwide problem affecting 35 million people. In the United States, almost two million people are affected by severe dementia, and another almost five million have milder forms of memory loss. High blood pressure caused by salt intake increases the risk of dementia by *six*, that is six *hundred* percent, not six percent. This information alone should be enough to make you throw away your saltshaker.

How about osteoporosis, which is referred to as the "silent

thief"? About 10 million Americans have osteoporosis and another 24 million have low bone mass, a precursor to osteoporosis. The number of hip fractures, wrist fractures and spinal fractures tops 1.25 million each year. These fractures cause severe suffering and long-term disability. About a quarter of hip fracture patients die in the very first year due to multiple complications. You can drop the prevalence of osteoporosis by as much as 30 percent simply by avoiding salt in your diet.

Let's look at stomach cancer, the second most common cause of cancer death worldwide, with nearly 800,000 reported cases per year. It is the number one cause of cancer death in countries like Japan, Korea, China and 39 different populations in 24 different countries. The research shows that salt intake significantly contributes to stomach cancer. The higher the salt intake, the higher is the likelihood of stomach cancer.

How big is the problem of obesity in America? Almost 30 percent of Americans are overweight. You do the math. We're not talking about looks here. Putting on pounds increases the risk of all these health problems many times over. No big secret. What many of us don't realize, however, is that the more salt you add to your food, the more you eat. All those unnecessary calories compromise your health.

Then comes asthma, which has become a very common problem among children in America. There are 22 million children in the United States affected by asthma; in addition, almost one in three people of Latino descent suffers likewise. Add salt to your diet and you are going to have more acute asthma attacks triggered by activity.

Lastly, salt consumption is a very big contributor for cardiovascular disease. In 2006, data from the Centers for Disease

Control (www.cdc.gov) shows that 850,000 Americans died of heart disease and strokes in that year alone. Let's think about this number for a moment: 850,000 lives lost in one year? Unfortunately, the story gets much worse. There are 16 million Americans living with heart disease. Once you have been diagnosed with heart disease, your life is changed forever. Some of the other grim statistics to consider: of the 785,000 Americans who had their first heart attack in 2006, 470,000 had a second or third heart attack the same year. This data does not even include the number of people affected by heart failure, which is the number one reason for admission to the hospital among Americans 65 years and older.

The data about strokes is just as alarming. In 2006, 137,000 Americans died of stroke. The actual number of stroke victims was 795,000, of whom 185,000 had their second or subsequent stroke.

By the way, the World Health Organization (WHO) has declared cardiovascular disease to be the number one killer worldwide, not just in America.

When you add all this up, we are talking about millions upon millions of people who are prematurely killed or maimed by salt intake. A series of scientific papers also sponsored by WHO and stemming from many prominent universities worldwide has shown exactly that. In any discussion about causes of preventable health problems, smoking usually takes the top spot. Smoking harms millions across the globe; therefore, smoking has been at the number one position among preventable causes of cardiovascular health problems for many decades.

Smoking still remains a huge problem, but new information about salt reveals that the number of deaths that could be reduced by mere salt reduction exceeds the number of lives that could be saved if people quit smoking. In one of the most telling publications, again sponsored by WHO, the number of deaths that could be avoided in a 10-year period worldwide is estimated at 13.8 million. This number still does not include the figures for disability and dysfunction, which would be several times that number.

What is the big difference if we name salt enemy number one or enemy number 100?

Let us compare how we as a society respond to these different catastrophic human problems. Acts of terrorism or a tsunami are not under the control of an individual, but salt intake is. Aren't we way too lackadaisical about a much larger problem affecting human lives? If you know who your primary enemy is, you will run away from it as fast as you can to safer ground, just like the tsunami victims did. If you are a parent, you will do the best you can to protect your children from that enemy. And if you are a government, you will pool all your resources to hunt down your most important enemy, just as in the case of Osama bin Laden.

Let's get rid of enemy number one in our food: salt.

Research

The urgent need to reduce sodium consumption

Havas S et al. 2007. Journal of the American Medical Association 298(12):1439–1441.

American Medical Association

- Worldwide, 16.7 million people die due to cardiovascular disease.
- About 26 percent of worldwide population has high blood pressure.
- Annual deaths from cardiovascular disease in USA: 850,000.
- Prehypertension, defined as BP greater than 120/80 and less than 140/90 mm Hg affects 27 percent of the population.
- Lifetime probability of having high blood pressure is 90 percent.
- Processed foods contribute to 77 percent of salt consumption in the U.S.

The authors issue a "call for action" to reduce salt intake. They cite the potential prevention of 150,000 deaths. Also discussed are the efforts by the AMA to get the FDA to remove salt from "Generally Accepted As Safe" (GRAS) status.

Projected effect of dietary salt reductions on future cardiovascular disease

Bibbins-Domingo K et al. 2010. New England Journal of Medicine 362:590–599.

University of California San Francisco, Stanford University, and Columbia University

American Heart Association and NIH

Using the Coronary Heart Disease policy model, projected health benefits are calculated. Reducing salt consumption by only 3 g/day from current levels of 15 to 20 g/day would accomplish the following benefits:

- New cases of coronary artery disease in U.S. reduced in the range of 60,000 to 120,000 per year.
- Number of strokes reduced in the range of 32,000 to 66,000 per year.
- Heart attacks reduced in the range of 44,000 to 99,000 per year.
- Annual deaths from any cause reduced in the range of 44,000 to 92,000 per year.
- Savings of 194,000 to 392,000 quality life years.
- Health care cost savings of $10 billion to $24 billion per year.
- In a 10-year period, 1 g/day salt reduction would be more cost effective than medications in all persons with high blood pressure.

Health benefits that can be realized by further reductions of salt intake would be many times greater.

Reducing population salt intake worldwide: from evidence to implementation

He FJ, MacGregor GA. 2010. Progress in Cardiovascular Diseases.

Queen Mary University, London, U.K.

The authors, who have extensively contributed to the body of information on the health problems of salt consumption, make the following observations:

- High blood pressure is responsible for 62 percent of strokes and 49 percent of coronary artery disease.
- Cumulative evidence comes from ecological findings, population studies, prospective cohort studies and outcome trials.
- Salt consumption is linked to several other health problems including obesity, left ventricular hypertrophy, osteoporosis, asthma severity, and stomach cancer.

The authors encourage a worldwide action plan to reduce salt consumption in order to achieve benefits in a very large area of health problems.

Chronic disease prevention: health effects and financial costs of strategies to reduce salt intake and control tobacco use

Perviz Asaria et al. 2007. Lancet 370:2044–53.

Kings Fund, London, U.K.; University of Auckland, Auckland, N.Z.; World Health Organization (WHO); Harvard School of Public Health, Boston, U.S.

The authors published a series of well-known papers about chronic diseases. This particular paper calculates (using WHO risk assessment protocol) the health impact of reduction of salt intake and tobacco use. According to WHO's database, cardiovascular disease has emerged as the number one cause of death and disability worldwide.

Over a 10-year period, 13.8 million deaths are determined to be avoidable, 75 percent of them from cardiovascular disease.

Reduction in salt intake is calculated to have the most impact in reducing these avoidable deaths worldwide—more so than reduction of tobacco use.

In addition, intervention to reduce tobacco use is more difficult and expensive, largely because of addiction to tobacco.

These findings lead the researchers to state: "Salt is enemy number one."

For more information
about salt and other health-related issues,
please visit healthnowbooks.com.

Chapter

High Blood Pressure

Salt, the newly crowned enemy number one, causes high blood pressure. By now you are probably assuming that adding salt to your food is just about the only reason anybody develops high blood pressure. Let us find out for sure. What is the evidence to connect salt to high blood pressure?

High blood pressure is *not* just a benign, pain-in-the-neck type of pesky issue that everybody seems to get sooner or later. What happens after you develop high blood pressure as you continue to add salt to your food? What are all the damaging affects of high blood pressure in the multiple organ systems of the human body? Once you are convinced of the salt = high blood pressure equation, you will find answers to all these questions.

And finally, why do certain sections of the population need extra protection from the salt habit? We'll review these special concerns. But first, let's look at the proof behind the assertion that once you add salt to your food, there is no escaping getting high blood pressure and all the problems that follow.

The Evidence

The International Federation and Society of Cardiology convened a multinational study called INTERSALT to answer the question, "What is the connection of adding salt to our food to developing high blood pressure?" This massive study involved over 10,000 people from 52 population groups from 32 countries across the world. Multiple international organizations, including the National Institute of Health, participated in and supported this large study. The results were originally published in 1988. This information seems to have languished for almost a decade until it was revisited by a report from the Department of Epidemiology at Northwestern University of Chicago in 1997.

This review of the INTERSALT study, after very detailed analysis, confirmed the findings of the original study. Among thousands of people tested across the world in the INTERSALT study, the more salt you add to the food the higher was the blood pressure.

While the scientific community received this information with great enthusiasm, the Salt Institute, an industry trade organization that represents salt manufacturers, disputed the findings. The Salt Institute claimed the conclusions of the INTERSALT study were unwarranted and not based on the proper interpretation of the data.

To address this issue further, a randomized prospective study (see glossary) was designed, called Trials of Hypertension

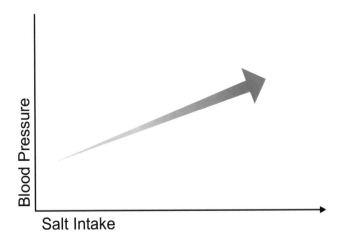

Blood Pressure

Salt Intake

Prevention (TOHP). This collaborative study involved Harvard, the National Institute of Health, the University of Pennsylvania, Johns Hopkins, and Loyola University Chicago. A total of 744 people at 10 different locations were studied for 18 months in TOHP I. In a second study, TOHP II, 2,383 people were studied for 36 months.

The conclusions and recommendations of this research were clear:

Salt has a direct causal relationship with high blood pressure.

These reports validated the findings of the INTERSALT Study. As far as the scientific community is concerned, the time has come to move past this argument and focus on how to educate people of this fact. Douglas Kamerow, the editor of the *British Medical Journal*, said it best: "Now that we have confirmed the connection between salt and high blood pressure, how do we convince people?"

Another editorial, titled "Time to Talk Salt," summarized the findings of these studies and said that this is the "final bugle call" in the battle of evidence. Many healthcare agencies and public health interest groups have also accepted these findings and their involvement has since accelerated.

In addition to confirming the findings of the INTERSALT study, the TOHP studies also found, when these patients were followed up after 15 years, a **25 percent reduction of cardiovascular deaths** correlated with a reduction in salt intake. We now know for sure that cutting salt in food reduces the chances of developing high blood pressure, and that translates into saving lives.

As with the TOHP studies, there are other significant findings from the INTERSALT study. A closer look at some of the groups among the 50 different populations enrolled in INTERSALT reveal further clues to the damage we do to ourselves in our love affair with salt. Yanomami Indians of the Brazilian jungles are one such population we can learn from.

Lessons from the Yanomami Indians

The Yanomami Indians are a tribe living in a very limited geographic area in the Brazilian Amazon jungles. During their entire history, they have never been exposed to salt and therefore never added salt to their diet. The only salt they consumed was what is naturally present in their food. The University of Rio de Janeiro published the findings on the Yanomami Indians in the INTERSALT study in 2003. Sophisticated tests performed on this population have confirmed the results of the INTERSALT study and revealed even more interesting findings.

1. If salt is never added to food from birth, adult blood pressure is likely to be 90/60 on average instead of 120/80, which is generally considered normal.

2. The blood pressure is likely to remain in the same range instead of increasing with advancing age.

3. Middle-age weight gain, which we take as part of the normal aging process, would not occur, either. The Yanomami Indians are one of a number of tribes who live in isolation without exposure to salt and who remain slender through advancing age.

Thus we have concluded from these investigations that salt intake indeed causes high blood pressure, and we have also seen some additional clues as to its harmful effects. There is no need for any further debate on whether salt consumption leads to high blood pressure. Instead, let us focus on learning more about high blood pressure and why we should try to prevent it (and what other damage comes from adding salt to our food).

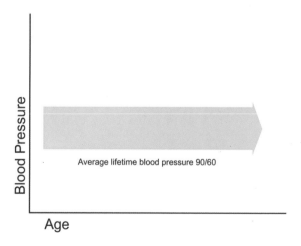

Yanomami Indians

Average lifetime blood pressure 90/60

Blood Pressure

Age

Young, Slender and Sleek   Older and Obese

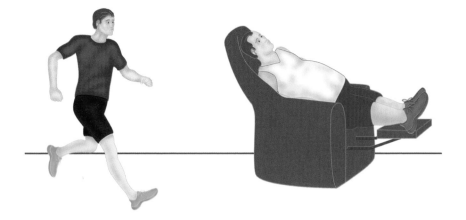

Research

INTERSALT: an international study of electrolyte excretion and blood pressure. Results for 24-hour urinary sodium and potassium excretion.

INTERSALT Cooperative Research Group. 1988. British Medical Journal 297; 319–328.

The INTERSALT Study: background, methods, findings, and implications

Stampler J. 1997. American Journal of Clinical Nutrition 65: S626–S642.

Department of Preventive Medicine, Northwestern University Medical School, Chicago, U.S.

The National Heart, Lung and Blood Institute (U.S.), The Wellcome Trust (U.K.), The International Society of Hypertension, The World Health Organization, The American Heart Association

Long term effects of dietary sodium reduction on cardio-vascular disease outcomes: observational follow-up of the trials of hypertension prevention (TOHP)

Cook NR et al. 2007. British Medical Journal 334:885–8.

Harvard Medical School, Boston, MA; National Heart, Lung, and Blood Institute, Bethesda, MD; University of Pennsylvania, Philadelphia, PA; Johns Hopkins University, Baltimore, MD; Loyola University, Maywood, IL

The Yanomami Indians in the INTERSALT Study

Jairo de Jesus Mancilha-Carvalho, Nelson Albuquerque de Souza e Silva. 2003.

Arquivos Brasileiros de Cardiologia 80:295–300.

From the Universidade Federal do Rio de Janeiro (FM/UFRJ)

For more information
about salt and other health-related issues,
please visit healthnowbooks.com.

Salt = High Blood Pressure

So we have learned from the Yanomami Indians and similar populations that, in almost all cases, if you never add salt to your food, your blood pressure is lower. Conversely, if you like to add salt to your food, you will have high blood pressure—guaranteed! You are born with plenty of sodium chloride—common table salt—without any need for adding more salt to your food. We do, however, need some salt. All the foods that we are naturally meant to consume provide us with just enough salt to meet this requirement.

Water makes up two thirds of our body with a number of different types of salts—called electrolytes—dissolved in it. Common everyday table salt can be found dissolved in many different types of bodily fluids. Complex mechanisms regulate the concentration of these electrolytes in the body very precisely.

Why should the concentration of common salt and other electrolytes in these fluids be maintained so precisely? To answer this question, let us look at blood, one of the most easily recognizable of body fluids. Blood actually gets its color from the red blood cells suspended in fluid called plasma. The red blood cells constantly travel in the blood vessels surrounded by the clear and colorless plasma. The salt concentration inside these red blood cells and the plasma all around them has to be kept exactly the same.

If the salt concentration in the plasma exceeds the salt concentration of the fluid inside the cells, some fluid from within the cells goes out into the surrounding fluid in an attempt to equalize the concentration. The cells, as a result, shrivel up and die.

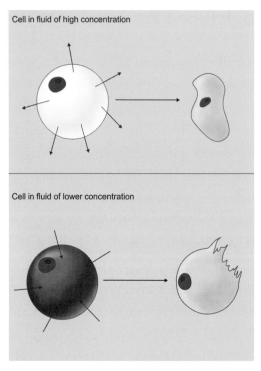

Cell in fluid of high concentration

Cell in fluid of lower concentration

If, on the other hand, the salt concentration in the red blood cells exceeds that of the surrounding fluid, then the fluid enters into the cells trying to equalize the concentration. Then, the cells swell up and eventually the cell walls burst. Therefore, the sum of all the dissolved contents inside the cells (electrolytes, or salts) must be equal to that of the liquid outside the cells in order to prevent any damage to the all-important cells.

Water that we would normally drink is never given intravenously in the hospital. Contact with pure water will damage the blood cells for reasons described above. Conversely, we cannot drink the saline (salty water) that is given to hospital patients intravenously in order to replace depleted body fluids. Attempting to drink this salt water will only induce vomiting, causing the body to lose even more water and electrolytes.

Adding more salt to what is naturally present in food, as we so commonly do, creates a problem for the very ingenious, complex mechanism our body uses to maintain the exact concentration of electrolytes. The kidneys maintain this crucial balance mainly by controlling the composition of urine. But, as it turns out, the kidney cannot completely get rid of all the excess salt we consume, especially over a long period of time.

To maintain the necessary balance between the fluid inside and outside the cells, the kidney compensates by retaining more water to make up for the excess salt not removed. Thus, the volume within the system increases, but the size of the system of blood vessels itself remains unchanged. The increased volume circulating in the unchanged system increases the pressure within the system (high blood pressure).

Consider the following example. You go on a vacation with a full suitcase. While there, you collect some souvenirs. Your overstuffed baggage cannot accommodate the new purchases. If you try, the pressure inside the bag and tension on the sides of the bag go up. To solve this problem, you would probably buy an extra bag so that everything fits easily. In the case of the human body, that option does not exist. You have only one vascular system, and its pressure will go up the more water you retain. 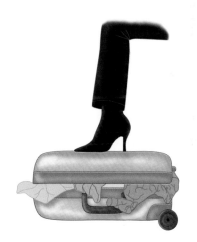 While there are many other complex mechanisms in play, the suitcase analogy is a good place to start, to understand why your love affair with salt makes your blood pressure go up.

Now that you understand the mechanism of high blood pressure from excess salt intake, we can move on to learning more about the health problems that result from high blood pressure.

Problems with High Blood Pressure

You just found out that you have high blood pressure, probably from all the years of adding salt to your food. So what? No big deal. Everybody around you has high blood pressure, too. Just take a few pills like all of your friends and family and everything will be fine! No, it does not work that way. There are so many dangerous problems with this all-too-common line of thinking. There are many serious consequences to having high blood pressure, and they cannot be fixed with a simple pill.

Diabetes, high cholesterol and high blood pressure are called "silent diseases" for a good reason. Until a really damaging event like a heart attack or stroke happens, they can remain unnoticed and undiagnosed. The main areas affected, referred to as "target organs," are the heart, the kidney, and the brain. High blood pressure, diabetes, high cholesterol and obesity are also interrelated. For example, one who has diabetes will often

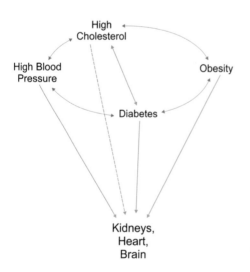

have blood pressure, obesity, and high cholesterol, and the overweight one will frequently have high blood pressure, diabetes and high cholesterol, and so on. Only aggressive surveillance can identify them at an early stage. It is also important to remember that high blood pressure and diabetes cannot be cured once they strike. Can you keep high blood pressure under control? Maybe.

Even when detected early, most people don't start treatment soon enough. During this delay, the silent damage to the target organs keeps on going. Furthermore, even after treatment has begun, often people don't take the pills as they are supposed to. The data on compliance to medications shows that when you have to take just one pill a day, you take it as directed only 60 percent of the time. And when you have to take a second pill, chances of taking both of them correctly drops to 30 percent. Most people with high blood pressure end up with at least three pills. You can just about forget taking the pills correctly as your main strategy to control these health problems.

Let us say you do take your pills on schedule, day in and day out. Your problems are not over yet. The way medications control blood pressure does not follow the same natural pattern of variation of blood pressure during the course of the day. Blood pressure normally changes from morning to afternoon, from afternoon to evening. There are differences in blood pressure from a sleeping to a waking state. In addition, the blood pressure is generally higher when you are in the doctor's office due to stress or nervousness. We call that "White Coat Syndrome."

TRIPLE FAILURE

Failure to detect early
Failure to start treatment early
Failure to take medications properly

Once you start medications, the blood pressure may still be above normal when resting and at the same time too low for physical activities. The body needs a certain level of blood pressure during physical activity. As a result of lower blood pressure from pills, most people experience a loss of energy and become less active. Reduced activity leads to weight gain. Increased weight in turn leads to higher blood pressure, thus setting up a vicious cycle. If the blood pressure remains high during the sleeping state, the cardiovascular damage continues in spite of swallowing multiple pills.

You also have to consider the cost of these multiple pills. Prescriptions can get expensive, and at this point you are trying to control more than one health problem. See what your salt habit is going to cost you! And let us not forget the side effects of many pills. More pills are added to control these side effects. What starts out as one or two pills ends up, for most people, becoming a whole bowl of pills in a fairly short time.

So there are many, many reasons why you should do all you can—especially cutting salt—to avoid any of these diseases. Your golden years should not be all about a bowl of pills, limited physical capabilities, lots of doctor's visits and many surgical procedures. Once you start treatment for one of these chronic ailments, such as high blood pressure, your life has to change forever anyway. Guess what? Now you also have to change what you eat. You will be forced to avoid eating things you love to eat. Pay attention to the salt in your food before any of these dreaded health problems take root. You can save yourself a lot of grief and have a more meaningful final third of your life by simply cutting salt in your food right now.

Special Considerations for African Americans

The addition of salt to our daily food, while not healthy for anybody, is downright horrible for African/Black Americans. Let's explore this problem starting with the following real-life scenario.

The phone rings at three in the morning. The nurse on the phone from the ICU apologetically says, "I am sorry to wake you up, Doc. I cannot get the blood pressure of this post-surgery patient under control." She goes on, "I know you are worried about bleeding problems after his heart surgery. I have already used the maximum doses of three different medications. I am still not able to bring down the blood pressure." I then give additional orders and hope the pressure comes down. Still concerned, I try to go back to sleep.

This conversation highlights the problem African Americans face in dealing with salt-induced high blood pressure. Data gathered from prominent sources such as the American Heart Association reveal that blacks have at least two times higher risk of high blood pressure than their Caucasian counterparts.

Hypertension in Blacks
• **Earlier age**
• **Higher BP**
• **More difficult to control**
• **More complications**

African Americans also have high blood pressure at an earlier age. The degree of the problem is also higher, meaning they suffer a higher rate of complications from a similar degree of high blood pressure. They require a stronger combination of medications, in spite of which, the blood pressure does not come under control, just like this patient we are taking care of above.

Among blacks, the risk of high blood pressure goes up even more with obesity, inactivity and diabetes, all of which are also unfortunately more common in African Americans compared to Caucasians. After finishing my first surgery one morning, there was a request for consultation waiting for me. I then go to see a young black lady—only 30 years old—with two beautiful children at her bedside. She needs an operation to make a connection between an artery and a vein (called a shunt) that can be easily accessed to perform dialysis. Her kidney failed during the birth of her last child three years ago. She has been dealing with very high blood pressure first diagnosed when she was 20.

> ## Hypertension in Blacks: Complications
> - **Stroke death increased four times**
> - **Heart disease increased three times**
> - **Heart failure risk doubled**
> - **Renal failure increased three times**

A 30-year-old person is not supposed to be hooked up to a machine every other day for several hours for the rest of her life. Isn't she going to miss enjoying the growing phases of her children, to say the least? Moreover, these dialysis shunts fail on a regular basis. She will end up needing so many more surgeries; shunt on this wrist, shunt on the other wrist, shunt in the forearm, shunt in the upper arm, on and on. Then you start revising this shunt and that shunt; the story never ends. What a life. What would you give not to be in that situation?

At the beginning of my career, I was considering specializing in this field just for the challenge of constructing vascular shunts. Dealing with this type of heartbreaking story day in day out, though, I found I could not stomach it, especially after I had my first child. Since then, I have developed a healthy respect for those who choose to handle the problems of kidney failure and dialysis.

Black Americans with high blood pressure suffer three times higher risk of renal failure. End stage renal failure requiring dialysis is a serious problem among blacks. Those who have high blood pressure are four times more likely to end up on dialysis in addition to the risk of heart attacks and heart failure.

Salt-induced high blood pressure causes another severely disabling problem: stroke. Among African Americans, the risk of having a stroke also runs very high, estimated at a staggering rate, four times that of Caucasians. Survivors of a stroke live with as much difficulty as anyone on dialysis. The inability to use an arm or a leg or both, and the inability to talk are only some of the gut-wrenching problems a stroke leaves you to live with.

Salt-induced high blood pressure can be prevented so that you don't have to face these serious problems. Based on all this well-documented data, African Americans should be much more aggressive in cutting salt from their diet.

Salt and Children

Adding salt is terrible for some populations but bad for everybody. Therefore, whether you belong to a population at a higher risk from salt intake or not, you should practice avoiding adding salt to your food at the earliest age possible. Although most of the diseases from excess salt intake show up later in life, you are sowing the seeds of these incurable diseases in infancy if you are adding any salt to your baby's food. You sow the seeds and keep nurturing them by continuing to add salt to their food as they grow. You want to promote the healthy growth of your child. The beautiful flowering plant of life is what you want but you are promoting the weed of disease that will later choke the healthy plant. You should never start adding salt to their or to your food. Why do you want to start something that they will have to stop later in order to stay healthy?

Let us review the basis for this tough stand. Salt-induced health problems, the ugly weed, are now showing up at a much younger age. In most industrialized countries, the health status of children is actually declining where it should be the opposite. If you haven't noticed, obesity runs rampant (almost one

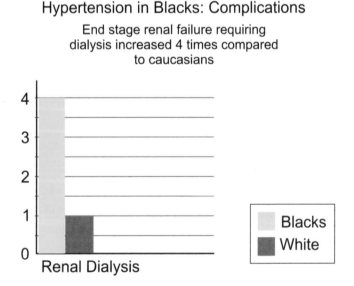

Hypertension in Blacks: Complications

End stage renal failure requiring
dialysis increased 4 times compared
to caucasians

in three) among children. Salt is a leading player in this tragedy. Some of the most common salty foods are actually empty calories. Consuming unnecessary salt and calories is a double whammy, or a one-two knock-out punch. No wonder childhood obesity has become such a big problem.

Along with excess pounds, high blood pressure and diabetes, even fat buildup in the arteries can be seen frequently among teenagers. Adding salt to food has a lot to do with every one of these problems.

It doesn't take very long for the excess salt in our food to show its damaging effects. The University of Melbourne reports a jump in blood pressure by a whopping one third among chimpanzees fed a high-salt diet for a mere 20 months. Humans share an almost 99 percent genetic match with chimps, which makes the findings of this landmark study very eye-opening.

Taking a cue from the studies on animals, research focusing on children has identified the same problems associated with adding salt to the food. In a report from St George's University of London, blood pressure steadily increased in proportion to salt intake among children age 4 to 18 years.

The research at Erasmus University, Netherlands, focused on children under the age of one year (neonates). In just six months, the babies placed on a low salt diet had a lower blood pressure. Not surprisingly, these children continue to have lower blood pressure even 15 years later. The blood pressure among populations never exposed to salt as seen earlier in the INTERSALT study was indeed lower (90/60). These findings make a very strong case for not adding salt from the very beginning of life.

Summarizing thirteen different studies among children,

another report from St. George's University of London concludes that the drop in blood pressure from not adding salt in infancy will dramatically reduce blood pressure and cardiovascular health problems as the children grow older.

It should be very clear by now that you should implement "no added salt" right from the very first time you start feeding your newborn. If you don't, you are guilty of planting, cultivating and nurturing the seeds for a multitude of health problems your baby will have to face later in life.

Research

The effect of increased salt intake on blood pressure of chimpanzees

Denton D et al. 1995. Nature Medicine 1:1009–1016.

Howard Florey Institute of Experimental Physiology & Medicine, University of Melbourne, Australia

Among the animal studies that have demonstrated the relationship of salt and high blood pressure, this publication is often quoted.

Chimpanzees have 98.8 percent genetic homology (similarity) with humans.

This is a randomized prospective study with 26 chimpanzees divided into two groups.

Study period: 20 months.

One group was fed a diet with salt intake of 0.5g/day (similar to salt intake of pre-agricultural revolution humans).

The second group was fed a diet with salt intake progressively increased to 15g/day (similar to salt intake of present-day adolescents).

Results: The blood pressure in the salt group was 33/10 mmHg higher than the low salt group by the end of only 20 months.

This study thus provided compelling evidence of the relationship of salt consumption to high blood pressure.

Salt and blood pressure in children and adolescents

He FJ et al. 2007. Journal of Human Hypertension.

St. George's University of London, London, U.K.

In this observational study, 1,658 children between 4 and 18 were studied for the relationship of their salt intake and blood pressure.

The study found that high blood pressure was related to salt intake in these children, and the higher the salt intake, the higher the blood pressure.

Long-term effects of neonatal sodium restriction on blood pressure

Geleijnse JM et al. 1997. Hypertension. 29:913–917.

Erasmus University Medical School, Rotterdam, Netherlands

The authors conducted a randomized double-blind controlled study on 476 newborn babies to test the impact of salt intake in early infancy on high blood pressure.

At the conclusion of the six-month trial, the low-salt group had a lower blood pressure. About 35 percent of the original participants were able to be tested 15 years later. The blood pressure was still lower after 15 years.

The authors concluded that the reduction of salt intake at birth has important long-term impact.

Importance of salt in determining blood pressure in children: meta-analysis of controlled trials.

He FJ, MacGregor GA. 2006. Hypertension 48:861–869.

St. George's University of London, London, U.K.

The authors conducted a meta-analysis of 13 different controlled trials involving children with regards to salt intake and high blood pressure. Three of these trials were in infants with

551 participants. The other ten trials included 966 participants with a mean age of 13 years. Mean duration of these trials was four weeks.

The authors found that even a modest reduction in salt intake at an early age has a significant impact in high blood pressure. The authors project this drop in blood pressure will drastically decrease cardiovascular disease in later years.

The authors therefore recommend aggressive reduction of salt intake at the earliest age.

> For more information
> about salt and other health-related issues,
> please visit healthnowbooks.com.

Chapter

The Heart and Blood Vessels

Salt-induced high blood pressure hurts the heart and blood vessels surprisingly in many different ways. In this chapter you will find out the extent of all these problems. Each one of these damaging effects is explained in simple language. Unique illustrations are used to help you better understand the mechanism of how adding salt to your food eventually leads to these health problems.

The Scenic Drive

The phone rings in the operating room. It is one of our cardiologists in the cath lab who wants to discuss a problematic situation. Fortunately, I am at a point in my surgery when I can take a moment to review his problem. The cardiologist says he has been working on a patient on the cath table for several hours, trying to open one of the blocked arteries with a balloon.

He found his patient's arteries to be very tortuous. "I have tried every catheter and guide wire available to me over and over," he says. "I cannot reach the actual location of the blockage in the artery, much less try to put in the balloon." The nurse pulls up the pictures on the computer in the operating room. After reviewing the pictures of the arteries, I advise the cardiologist on the intercom to conclude the procedure. The balloon procedure, as a choice of treatment, is eliminated for this patient. It's impossible. We have to re-evaluate him to see whether he can be treated with medicines only or whether he is a candidate for bypass surgery. Either way, this patient's future quality of life will be severely compromised.

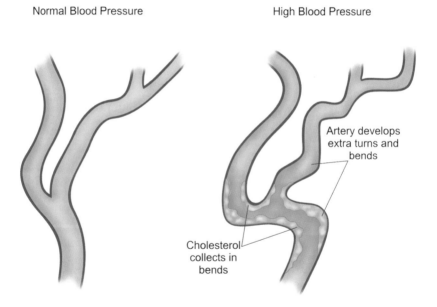

Normal Blood Pressure

High Blood Pressure

Artery develops
extra turns and
bends

Cholesterol
collects in
bends

This event reminds me of a recent trip to the West Coast. We visited our family friends in Thousand Oaks, California, a northern suburb of Los Angeles. We were planning to fly back from Los Angeles International Airport, which is to the south. The fastest and shortest way is to take Highway 101 and exit to highway 405 southbound. Traffic conditions, however, can change this entire plan. Our host suggested an alternate route, since we had some time to spare. We took the Malibu Canyon Road, which is a very winding scenic drive through the hills, and ended up on Pacific Coast Highway at the entrance to Pepperdine University. Going south along the coastline of the famous Malibu Beach, Santa Monica, etc., we took Lincoln Road to the airport. It was a very, very scenic route indeed.

There is a big difference in the traffic flow between these two roads to the airport. On a scenic drive, you cannot drive the same speed as a highway. At each one of the bends and turns, you have to slow down and have your foot on the brakes. Otherwise, you will run off the road.

If you have the time, a leisurely drive along a meandering road is fun. Unfortunately, the reverse is true when it comes to our bodies. High blood pressure over time turns arteries, which start out more like highways, into winding drives. Frequently, there are steep bends like hairpin turns. The blood is flowing through these twisting arteries the same way, actually at an even higher pressure. So at every turn and bend of the artery, as you can imagine, there are quite a lot of shearing forces in play. This fight between the flowing blood and the wall of the artery is going on with each heartbeat. In due time, the inside lining of the arteries is damaged at all these friction points.

Cholesterol is prone to deposit wherever there is damage to the inside lining of the arteries. These deposits eventually block the flow of blood. Just as with the patient in the cath lab, you cannot always navigate these crooked and clogged arteries with wires and catheters.

More than 90 percent of people in America and worldwide are expected to have high blood pressure. Ironically, it is easy to avoid high blood pressure and all the complications it creates. Adding salt to your diet is just about the only reason to develop high blood pressure. And sooner or later, everybody who adds salt to his or her food will develop high blood pressure.

Once you have fat buildup in your arteries, you may have to go through a horrific surgery such as coronary artery bypass. But if your arteries take a scenic drive, the surgery will be more difficult to accomplish. You may also lose the option of a common procedure to open the blockage with a balloon. Therefore, cut down the salt in your diet so that your arteries don't take a scenic drive (see illustration). If you don't take kicking this salt habit seriously, you are in double jeopardy: not only will you build cholesterol in your arteries, you will be left with more difficult choices of treatment for the eventual and inevitable fat buildup in the arteries.

Fat Deposits in My Arteries?

Whenever I take the fat from inside an artery during surgery, I make it a point of saving it and then showing it to the patient and family. "Oh my God! Is that what you took out of my artery?" says the typical patient who gets to see the specimen I removed in order to clean a clogged artery. The ugly irregular-looking piece of fat catches their attention every time. It is hard as a rock and rattles as I shake the bottle. There are pieces of fresh clot in some of the many crevices in the surface ready to break loose. Even though I always show my patients photographs of cholesterol deposits before they ever go into surgery, they are shocked when they see the real thing that has come out of their own bodies. You should see their stunned faces. "I would have never believed it if you had not shown it to me," says the patient of the life-threatening deposit.

The colossal irony is that they could have avoided this whole situation in the first place. Fat does not need to be depositing in the wall of any blood vessels. But that's exactly what's happening over and over again in millions of peo-

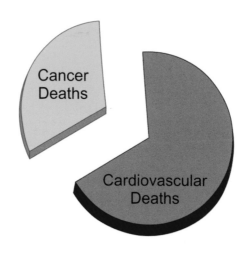

ple. Cardiovascular disease that comes from fat buildup in the arteries of the heart and blood vessels all over the body is *the* number one killer of people around the world. If you combine deaths from every known cancer, the most commonly feared disease of all, it doesn't add up to the number killed by cardiovascular disease.

Counting deaths is only part of the total picture of the damage from fat buildup in the arteries. These days, we are doing a much better job taking care of the people dealing with the consequences of this fat buildup. As a result, the number of people alive but disabled from cardiovascular disease now runs in the millions and millions, many times more than the actual deaths. What an alarming fact.

Carotid Surgery

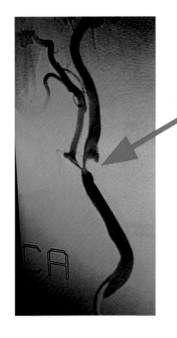

Cholesterol in the artery in the neck.

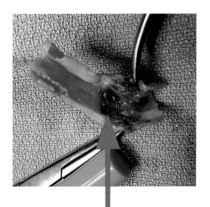

Cholesterol from the same artery. Note the irregular surface, ulceration and clot.

Sadly, we are hardly making any progress in the prevention of cardiovascular disease. Consequently, an ever-increasing pool of people who represent a big section of the population now live with disability and dysfunction.

As we take care of these people, one cannot help but reflect: We are improving life expectancy, but are we improving health?

Are we actually prolonging life? Or are we simply prolonging the process of death? And why aren't we focusing more on prevention, since, ironically, this self-inflicted death and disability from cholesterol buildup in the arteries can largely be prevented? To understand how we can prevent cardiovascular disease, we must first understand how and why cholesterol builds in the arteries. Arteries are a network of tubes carrying blood from the heart to all over the body. With each beat, the heart pumps more blood into the arteries. The walls of these arteries have a certain amount of "give" to accommodate the flow in synchrony with the heartbeat. Much like two long-time dancing partners moving gracefully in synchrony with each other, the heart and the blood vessels function in a coordinated fashion. When one partner moves in, the other backs up just enough to compensate. If the dance partners are not in sync, they step on one another's toes and one or both can get hurt. Correspondingly, in our bodies as the blood pressure goes up, a fight begins between the wall of the artery and the higher pressure of the flow of blood. Like the toes of the out-of-sync dance partners, over time the inside lining of the artery falls victim. Damage begins where the arteries branch or make turns.

Once there are areas of damage to the inside lining of the arteries, fat starts to deposit in these locations. The walls of the arteries are not the normal location for fat storage. Food consumed in excess of the immediate requirements of the body gets stored as fat to be used for a rainy day. A baby, for example, has a lot of fat reserves (see picture). You see this fat stored in the cheeks, buttocks, belly, etc., but not in the walls of the arteries.

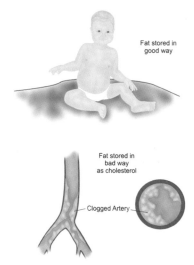

Fat stored in good way

Fat stored in bad way as cholesterol

Clogged Artery

Once cholesterol deposit

begins, it keeps rapidly increasing. Growing cholesterol deposits in the wall of the artery cause the path for bloodflow to become progressively smaller; eventually, it stops up altogether. Consequently, the most feared, unwelcome and well-known event, a heart attack, occurs when a portion of the heart muscle suddenly loses its blood supply in this way. A portion of the heart muscle actually dies from lack of oxygen.

Survival after any heart attack depends upon the amount of heart muscle lost. Sudden loss of a large part of the heart muscle is fatal. The pumping capability of the heart goes down with multiple smaller heart attacks. The most commonly known variety of heart failure comes from a number of these small heart attacks when small arteries get clogged with fat.

Cholesterol buildup affects arteries of many other parts of the body as well. Stroke, kidney failure, and loss of circulation to the legs, etc., are some of the other well-known consequences of blocked arteries. For example, when an artery carrying blood to the brain is clogged, you get a stroke much like a heart attack.

The wall of a larger artery such as the aorta sometimes becomes weak from cholesterol buildup. As the blood is flowing through this artery continuously under pressure, the weak part of the arterial wall begins to expand (see illustration). This weak, expanded or bulged area of the artery, called an aneurysm, can have deadly consequences. Once

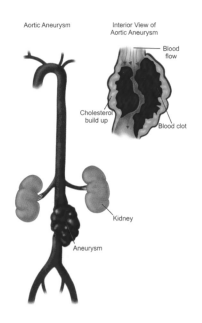

Aortic Aneurysm

Interior View of
Aortic Aneurysm

Blood
flow

Cholesterol
build up

Blood clot

Kidney

Aneurysm

this aneurysm grows to a certain size, it will rupture. The blood inside the arterial system suddenly escapes out of it and death from blood loss comes rather quickly. Salt-induced high blood pressure contributes to the stretching of the aorta from cholesterol buildup as well as to the rupture event itself.

Adding salt to our food is a major contributor of fat (cholesterol) buildup in the arteries. We know salt-induced high blood pressure doubles the risk of this biggest cause of death and disability around the world. So if your salt habit doesn't kill you prematurely from fat buildup in your arteries, you are for sure looking at spending almost a third or more of your later life with some disability and dysfunction.

If you don't care about what your state of health does to your family or what it costs society, at least you should care about what you are doing to yourself. You absolutely don't want any fat building up in your arteries. Once this realization dawns, you will begin to dislike the taste of salt in your food, since placing your trust in any pill or surgical procedure is not as helpful as simply avoiding excess salt. Loss of heart muscle from multiple small heart attacks from fat buildup leading to heart failure is in your future if you don't heed this advice.

My Heart Is Failing

Why are so many Americans—actually over a million—being admitted to the hospital each year with "heart failure"? Among Americans 65 or older, heart failure has become the number one reason for hospitalization. More than five million Americans are affected, and every year 250,000 of them do not make it out of the hospital. To assess this rapidly growing nationwide problem, the National Institute of Health (NIH) sponsored a database named ADHERE, short for Acute Decompensated Heart Failure.

More than 200,000 patients from 275 hospitals in America were enrolled by the end of the study period. Once you wake up to the relationship between salt intake and high blood pressure, the information from this massive database is essential to understanding the damage we inflict on our own heart by salt-induced high blood pressure.

Doctors use the term "heart failure" when a patient's heart cannot pump enough blood to keep up with the usual needs of the body. Don't compare it with light bulb failure or car engine failure. In the early stages, the signs of heart failure are very subtle. Decrease in the ability to do some of the activities that one could perform previously is the earliest sign. In the advanced stage requiring hospitalization (decompensated), you can't tolerate even minimal activity. At this stage you will notice swelling of the feet and shortness of breath at rest or with minimal daily activity. Once in the hospital, after a few days of treatment, the severe symptoms improve (compensated) and you go home, but only for the time being.

Soon enough, the symptoms worsen and you end up in the hospital again. With each successive hospitalization it becomes more difficult to control the heart failure, and the need for hospitalization becomes more frequent. Once heart failure starts, only half of the affected people survive five years—with a lot of medications and frequent hospitalizations. One third of the people admitted with heart failure do not survive beyond one year.

Heart failure conventionally is thought of as the result of loss of the heart muscle due to heart attacks caused by cholesterol build up. The pumping cycle of the heart has two phases. The systole is when heart muscle squeezes to pump the blood. The diastole is the phase when the heart muscle relaxes to fill with blood to be pumped. The loss of heart muscle from heart attacks reduces the pumping ability, the systolic function of the heart, leading to heart failure. ADHERE has found that in half the patients admitted in this registry, the systolic function is not affected. Overgrowth of the heart muscle from long-standing high blood pressure decreases the *relaxing* ability of the heart muscle, causing diastolic dysfunction.

Diastolic dysfunction, by itself without any systolic dysfunction, is responsible for an astonishing 50 percent of the admitted population in this registry. This is a major eye opener, bringing into focus the devastating impact of diastolic dysfunction.

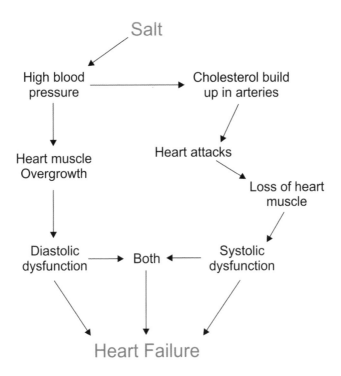

Combining the information from very large population-based databases such as INTERSALT and ADHERE, we can see the effects of salt consumption. Salt consumption will lead to high blood pressure, and high blood pressure leads to enlargement of the heart as well as increasing the risk of cholesterol buildup in the arteries of the heart. Heart attacks result in systolic dysfunction and heart muscle overgrowth leads to diastolic dysfunction.

Cut salt from your food so you can get off this road that leads to heart failure, one way (systolic dysfunction) or another (diastolic dysfunction).

Lessons from ADHERE

1. Five million Americans affected.
2. 500,000 new cases each year.
3. 250,000 heart failure patients die each year.
4. Death from heart failure is 33 percent within the first year.
5. Readmission to the hospital is 50 percent in six months.
6. With each readmission, function ability rapidly keeps going down.
7. The systolic (pumping) cycle of the heart is not damaged in half the people hospitalized with heart failure.

Research

Acute Decompensated Heart Failure National Registry

www.clinicaltrials.gov/ct2/show/NCT00366639

ADHERE Scientific Advisory Committee and Investigators

From the Division of Cardiovascular Medicine, Ohio State University, Columbus, Ohio; Division of Cardiology, University of North Carolina at Chapel Hill, Chapel Hill, North Carolina; Ahmanson-UCLA Cardiomyopathy Center, University of California, Los Angeles Medical Center, Los Angeles, California; Midwest Heart Specialists, Naperville, Illinois; Heart Failure Program, Hackensack University Medical Center, Hackensack, New Jersey; Cardiology Division, Albert Einstein College of Medicine, New York; and Scios Inc., Fremont, California.

This study was funded by Scios, Inc., and sponsored by NIH.

For more information
about salt and other health-related issues,
please visit healthnowbooks.com.

Atrial Fibrillation

While an overgrown heart muscle takes you down the road to heart failure, the same salt-induced high blood pressure also stretches the walls of the heart chambers. Damage to the electrical wiring that travels in the walls of the heart leads to a different problem.

Remember when President George H. Bush, the 41st President of the United States, (not George W.) nearly fainted at Camp David? The day, May 4, 1991, was probably when most Americans first heard the term "atrial fibrillation." The President was not having a heart attack, but his heartbeat was very fast and erratic. He was immediately taken to the hospital and placed on strong blood thinners and medications to control this fast, irregular heartbeat called atrial fibrillation. An overactive thyroid condition called Graves disease was responsible for the President's atrial fibrillation, but there is a strong connection to salt intake in most people who develop this condition.

High blood pressure from salt consumption makes the heart muscle grow big. The overgrown heart muscle does not relax well; it is also stiffer, which requires higher pressure to fill it. The atrial chambers of the heart that pump to fill the ventricles are subject to this increase in pressure. The atria, unlike the ventricles, are very thin walled. In response to the increasing pressure, the walls of the atria begin to stretch. The electrical wiring of the heart travels in the walls of the atrium just like in the walls of your house. The stretch injury disrupts this wiring. Independent, autonomous spots of heartbeats originate from multiple locations in these walls; when the walls stretch and the wiring gets damaged, the whole atrium is no longer beating as one and begins to quiver. That's fibrillation.

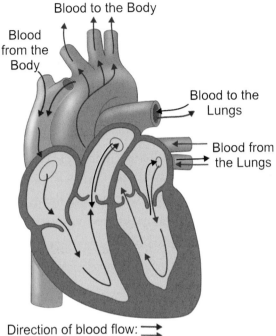

Blood to the Body

Blood from the Body

Blood to the Lungs

Blood from the Lungs

Direction of blood flow: ⇉
Reverse direction of increased filling pressure
in left ventricle: →

In a healthy heart, the chambers that receive the blood from the body and the lungs—the atria—start the beat by emptying the blood into the pumping chambers, the ventricles. The ventricles beat next in synchrony and pump the blood forward. Once A-fib develops, the rhythmic two-step cycle of the heartbeat is gone. The center that controls the heart rate (the number of heartbeats per minute) is also in the atrium. The heart rate normally changes with the demands of the body: the rate is slow during sleep and goes up in proportion to the activity. In atrial fibrillation, the walls of the chamber are no longer pumping; they are instead simply quivering rapidly (hence the name fibrillation).

The blood stagnates (pools) in some areas within the non-pumping atrial chambers. It is the nature of blood to clot when it is not flowing. These clots break loose from time to time and end up in different parts of the body. Arteries to the brain are among the very first branches from the heart. If the clot goes into one of these arteries to the brain, that is a stroke, hence the need for strong blood thinners in atrial fibrillation cases.

Once you are in A-fib you will be placed on strong blood thinners to prevent clots from forming in the heart. The blood thinner level has to be maintained in a certain narrow range. If it is too high, there can be major spontaneous bleeding problems. Stroke can also occur from spontaneous bleeding caused by an excess of blood thinner. If it is too low, clotting can go on. This is walking a tightrope. It is frustrating to the point where some doctors describe it as giving somebody a new disease in attempting to control another.

Blood thinners are not the only medication you will need. The fast and erratic heart rate has to be controlled. At a very fast rate, the heart does not pump out as much blood. The pumping action of the atria contributes up to 25 percent of the cardiac output, but this is lost in atrial fibrillation. The elderly are more likely to suffer this sudden loss of a quarter of the cardiac output. Normally, the heart rate is expected to fluctuate based on the activity level. In atrial fibrillation, your heart may still be going fast when you want to sleep, but it may be too slow for any brisk activity. A sudden shift in the normal heart rhythm to atrial fibrillation quickly drops the amount of blood pumped by the heart (cardiac output). President George H. Bush nearly fainted because of this sudden change in oxygenated blood supply to his brain.

Almost two million Americans are afflicted by A-fib—not just the former President. Heart failure is the most common reason for hospitalization once you are 65 years old or older, and atrial fibrillation is present a whopping 40 percent of the time. It is not as benign as you may have been led to believe. Nearly 75,000 strokes in America every year are attributed to atrial fibrillation. The elderly are more commonly affected. Putting it another way, almost a third of the strokes suffered by the elderly are a complication of atrial fibrillation. Any number of stroke victims and their families will tell you, this is worse than death. For example, a stroke on the left side of the brain leaves you without the ability to talk and a loss of function on the right side of the body. You cannot communicate, nor can you use your dominant hand. Just imagine that state. No wonder these victims are in such despair.

So don't add salt to your food if you want to avoid atrial fibrillation and the complications of its treatment. That is not all. There are severe consequences to the enlarged heart that results from the ongoing fight with high blood pressure.

I Have a Big Heart

High blood pressure as a result of adding salt to your food has made your heart grow big. It is not a good thing to have your physical heart grow bigger than it should be. As the heart muscle pushes harder to deal with higher pressure in the vascular system, the heart is getting a workout, as though it were in a gym. This workout is going on with each and every heartbeat, day in and day out.

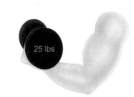

Over time, the heart muscle grows bigger, just like any other muscle working against increasing resistance, like lifting weights.

The big heart can still squeeze the blood forward (the systole part of the heartbeat cycle) just as before. Unfortunately, all the problems come from this overgrown heart muscle not being able to relax fully after each systole. Problems of this part of the heartbeat cycle—remember, it's called diastolic dysfunction—will lead to heart failure in many different ways.

Normal Heart Muscle

Enlarged Heart Muscle

The backswing

Take a look at the swing of a golfer to understand what happens to heart function when the heart cannot relax after pumping. The motion of the forward swing of the golfer and systole of the heart are similar. In preparation for the forward swing, the golfer takes the golf club back as far he can. The backswing is a very important part of the golfer's attempt to make the ball travel as far as possible.

This backswing and diastole of the heart are similar. How far the ball will travel depends upon the backswing as well as the forward swing. As the backswing becomes smaller and smaller, the distance you can hit the ball becomes shorter and

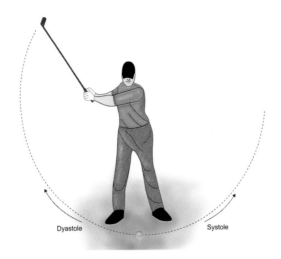

Dyastole   Systole

shorter. As the heart keeps getting bigger, the relaxing ability—which is like the golfer's backswing—is also getting shorter. The amount of blood sent to your body per heartbeat becomes less and less, just as the golf ball will go shorter and shorter distances with smaller and smaller backswings. Eventually, your heart cannot keep up with the requirements of daily activity—just from this loss of backswing—and you are in heart failure. Let's see in how many other ways this heart failure comes about from simply enlarging the heart.

Big heart but small capacity

The size of the pumping chamber also decreases with increasing thickness of the heart muscle (see illustration on next page). Before the heart pumps, the chamber has to fill up. The amount of blood pumped with each heartbeat depends upon the amount of volume in the chamber at the end of the filling phase. An enlarged heart pumps less blood with each heartbeat.

cardiac output = volume x heart rate.

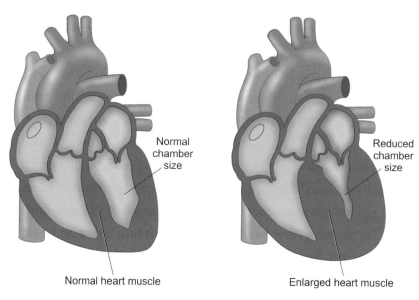

Normal chamber size

Reduced chamber size

Normal heart muscle

Enlarged heart muscle

So if the chamber size decreases, overall cardiac output also proportionately decreases. The heart compensates to a degree by increasing the heart rate. Beta blockers, one of the medications often given to control high blood pressure, work to protect the heart by reducing the heart rate. If you are on this medication, now the heart rate cannot go up to compensate for the decrease in chamber size, and you may not be getting enough blood pumped through your system. You could actually feel worse once you start taking pills to control high blood pressure! So decreasing the size of the pumping chamber of a big heart by itself can contribute to heart failure.

The baseball heart

The shape of the normal heart is changed from overgrowth of the heart muscle. The oval shape of the normal heart, like an American football, has a well-designed purpose. This football has a closed end and opens at the other. The walls of the heart

Normal Heart (shaped like a football)

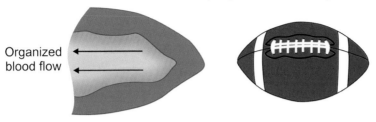

Organized
blood flow

Enlarged Heart (shaped like a baseball)

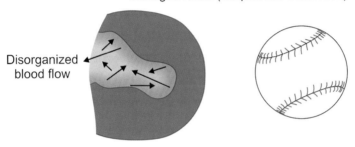

Disorganized
blood flow

chamber squeeze in a coordinated fashion to propel the blood through the open end into the vascular system.

The enlarged heart has changed its shape. Heart surgeons like me have described an enlarged heart for a long time as stiff and round, like a baseball. We have known for a long time now that these baseball hearts don't function well.

The walls of a baseball heart don't squeeze in the same coordinated fashion as a football. The forces of propulsion are working against each other instead of propelling in one direction toward the open end. Cardiac output of course will fall. Interestingly, you notice that your face had an oval shape when you were younger and slender. Now that you have added some pounds, the face has become more round. The same thing is going on with the heart muscle. A round and stiff baseball heart means less cardiac output and eventual heart failure.

I feel my heart pounding away

The heart is doing its thing, pumping blood constantly to keep up with the requirements of the body, but you are not aware of any of the heartbeats. You are not supposed to be. If you suddenly become aware of your heartbeat, you could have a dangerous type of irregular heartbeat from problems with the electrical system of the heart related to its blood supply.

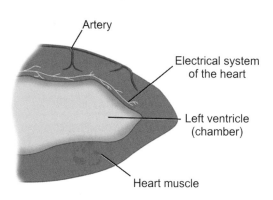

Artery

Electrical system of the heart

Left ventricle (chamber)

Heart muscle

The electrical system of the heart muscle travels in a space very close to the inside chamber of the heart. The arteries of the heart that carry blood to the heart muscle travel on the surface of the heart. These arteries send branches into the muscle, going through the muscle itself in a perpendicular way (see illustration). The muscle closest to the chamber is therefore the farthest point of blood supply.

This area is even further away in a heart that has enlarged from salt-induced high blood pressure. Another interesting factor: although the heart pumps blood to the body during the pumping phase (systole), the muscle itself receives blood only during the relaxing phase of the heart cycle (diastole). A stiff, thick heart takes a higher pressure to fill up. Because of this higher filling pressure in an enlarged heart, the muscle closest to the chamber (sub endocardium) is often at risk of critical loss of blood supply. The electrical system of the ventricles travels in this very same area. Small scars here create dangerous irregular heartbeats of the pumping chambers (ventricular arrhythmia).

Ventricular arrhythmia, unlike atrial arrhythmia, can be deadly. This abnormal rhythm can accelerate very quickly into cardiac arrest and sudden death. A special type of pacemaker designed to detect these irregular beats will deliver a shock to break this deadly rhythm. Because of the prohibitive cost of these devices, they can be placed only if the heart function has deteriorated beyond a certain point.

So watch out. If you become aware of your heartbeat, one of the deadliest of the complications from long-term salt intake could be upon you.

My valve leaks!

The heart actually has four different pumping chambers. There are four valves in the heart that open to allow the blood flow in one direction but close to prevent the flow in the reverse direction. The mitral valve, located between the left atrium and the left ventricle, prevents blood going back into the left

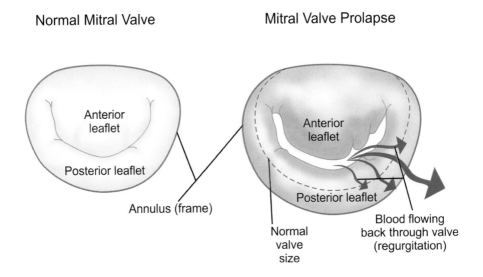

Normal Mitral Valve

Mitral Valve Prolapse

Anterior leaflet

Posterior leaflet

Annulus (frame)

Anterior leaflet

Posterior leaflet

Normal valve size

Blood flowing back through valve (regurgitation)

atrium when the left ventricle pumps blood forward into the body. This valve opens when the left ventricle is relaxing to fill with blood.

The mitral valve consists of two curtain-like structures, the leaflets, which are mounted on a frame inside the heart, called the annulus. These leaflets open and close with each and every pumping and relaxing cycle of the heart. They are like two doors mounted on a frame in the wall. As the heart muscle grows bigger and bigger in response to salt-induced high blood pressure, this frame (annulus) becomes wider. When the valve leaflets close while mounted on a wider frame, they cannot come together completely, leaving a gap in the middle. With each heartbeat, the left ventricle pumps and the blood leaks back into the left atrium through this gap.

The overgrown heart also damages the mitral valve in another way. Not only are the mitral valve leaflets attached to the annulus like doors on a frame, strong strings anchor the free edge to the heart muscle. These strings—called chordae tendinae—work like the strings of a parachute, holding the edges down. As the heart muscle grows, some of these strings are stretched. When one of these strings snaps from the stretch injury, the corresponding edge of the valve floats free. The edges of the valve do not come together at this location, leaving a gap when the left ventricle pumps. And again, blood leaks back into the left atrium with each heartbeat.

The pressure in the left atrium goes up from a leaky mitral valve and sets up a chain of events. The walls of the left atrium are thin and stretch. Atrial fibrillation comes from damaged electrical wiring in the walls of the left atrium. Feeling tired easily will be the earliest of the symptoms, but it may often be ignored as merely a sign of getting older. Later, as heart failure sets in, feeling short of breath with minimal activity, swelling of the feet, etc., will be noticed.

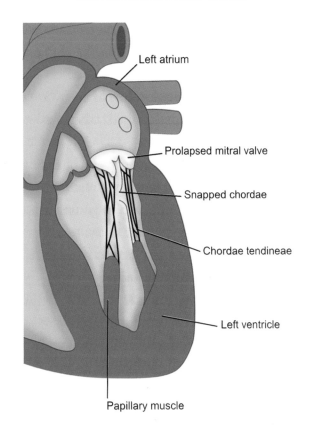

Surgery for a leaking mitral valve used to be a rare operation until a few years ago. Now it has become one of the most common heart surgeries performed in America. Surgery can fix a leaking mitral valve. It is a big operation. This surgery does not solve all other related problems of the big heart.

Thus there are many different ways the big heart resulting from excess salt in your food will lead to heart failure. Adding salt to food is so universal, no wonder millions and millions of Americans are dealing with heart failure. Once heart failure has set in . . . you know the rest of the story. Don't wait to cut salt in your food. Do it now so that you don't end up with a big failing heart.

Chapter

Not Just the Heart

There is a lot more bad news. The salt habit causes many other problems, not just heart problems. In this chapter, you will discover, for instance, the connection between salt intake and obesity, asthma and osteoporosis. Of even greater concern should be the risk of getting stomach cancer or memory loss from adding salt to your food.

Asthma

You may not believe this story, but it's true. In fact, I have heard similar stories from any number of people—family members, friends, patients, etc.

"There is something wrong with this telephone," complains a teenager. "It makes me go into an asthma attack. I get short of breath and start wheezing and coughing." She has done a lot of shopping for a new phone without much luck; they all seem to have the same problem.

There is nothing wrong with the phone itself. The real issue is that she has been living with asthma, which is triggered by her long phone conversations. Unfortunately, this is not uncommon for kids these days. You often see on television and at school games, kids using inhalers on the sidelines after a run. They are experiencing an exercise-induced asthmatic attack. As we saw in the young lady above, even a simple event like speaking long uninterrupted sentences can be enough to trigger such attacks.

Adding salt to your food is responsible for increasing the frequency of these exercise-induced asthma attacks. New research is clear: the more salt in your food, the higher the number of these attacks.

The lung looks like a kitchen sponge, full of small air cells. Each of these small air cells (alveoli) connects to the main breathing passage in the same way branches of a tree—all the way out to the leaves—connect to the main trunk. In asthma, the final branch leading to the leaf (bronchiole) is inflamed. Inflammation means swelling, and the swelling narrows the passage for air exchange (see illustration). Quick spasms of already swollen bronchioles close the passage, further triggering an acute asthmatic attack. We have already shown that adding salt to your food promotes fluid retention to maintain the balance of salt concentration in your body fluids. Swelling from this excess fluid around the small breathing passages is a set-up to trigger asthmatic attacks more easily. Water retention could also be responsible for excess mucus production, which contributes to blocking the airway as well.

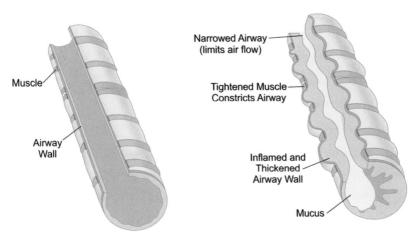

Narrowed Airway
(limits air flow)

Tightened Muscle
Constricts Airway

Muscle

Airway
Wall

Inflamed and
Thickened
Airway Wall

Mucus

Normal Airway

Airway With Asthma Symptoms

This young lady is but one example of millions (22 million, actually) of American children and teens who suffer from asthma. One in three children of Latin descent has asthma. These children go through multiple medications, inhalers and nebulizers for many years. The fear of triggering an attack can decrease the activity level in the formative years. The long-term impact of these medications and reduced activity has not been fully assessed, but common sense dictates that it cannot be good.

Have you ever experienced a situation when you simply cannot breathe, start wheezing and relentlessly cough your guts out? Have any of your family members—especially children—gone through these episodes? Then you will want to do all you can to cut down the chances of having one of these spells. Cut the salt in your diet and breathe easier.

Research

Dietary sodium intake and asthma: an epidemiological and clinical review

Mickleborough TD, Fogarty A. 2006. International Journal of Clinical Practice.

Indiana University

This research demonstrated that reducing salt intake for just two weeks alters airway inflammation. This is one of the major problems in asthma. The flow of oxygen into the bloodstream, termed the diffusion capacity of the lungs, is also affected.

In this study, the lung function improved and bronchial reactivity decreased with just two to five weeks of a low sodium diet, while sodium loading made it worse. Exercise-induced asthma also decreased by maintaining salt reduction only for one to two weeks.

Salt intake, asthma, and exercise-induced bronchoconstriction: a review.

Mickleborough TD. 2010 The Physician and Sportsmedicine. Apr. 38(1):118–31.

Indiana University

The authors reviewed all the published literature to date dealing with the connection of salt intake to asthma.

Based on this extensive review coupled with their own research, the author makes the following points.

1. A low salt diet decreases exercise-induced bronchospasm.
2. In the treatment of asthma, a low sodium diet can be considered a therapeutic option as an adjunct to medications.

Salt Makes Me Obese?

"Saturday Night Fever"! That was quite a movie when I first came to America. Remember John Travolta? Slim and slender, he moved across the dance floor with so much grace and vigor. People went to see this movie just to watch him and listen to the Bee Gee's music. Travolta was sensational, the talk of the town for several years. The image of his dance pose has been unforgettable. Have you seen any of the images of his body lately? He is not the same slim, slender person from that movie, is he? It is not likely that he can dance like that now.

But why pick on John Travolta? He is not the only one. You can think of many examples of this change among your own friends and family, and many celebrities. They all have put on quite a few pounds by the time they reached 40, and some even sooner. This so-called middle age weight gain has long been considered a normal part of aging. It is just like accepting that you cannot do the same physical activity as you did a decade or two ago and cannot remember as well as you used to. Putting on weight is a vicious cycle. As you gain pounds you become less active and put on more weight. We all know that once you put on weight, it very difficult to lose it.

The problem of obesity is not reserved for middle-aged people. Obesity affects Americans of all ages, including children. The Centers for Disease Control reports about 34 percent of all men and 36 percent of all women are obese. Nearly 20 percent of children and almost a third of teenagers are obese. Experts in the field of obesity say these numbers are actually conservative. If you look at the number of people whose body weight is within the ideal range for age and body frame, the problem of obesity is much worse. And there is a steady upward trend of obesity among all age groups.

Obesity is a major health problem facing America. It is not really about a person's appearance. There is plenty of evidence that obesity promotes diabetes, high blood pressure, heart disease, cancers, joint disease and more. And just like night follows day, those will curtail your life. Remember, many of these serious health problems are not curable. The best you can hope for is to control them. You will be on a long painful journey ending up eventually in premature death. Once you are afflicted with obesity-induced health challenges, you are alive but how well are you really living?

Adding salt to your food directly contributes to obesity in a very big way. This connection is very easy to explain. First, try to eat potato chips or peanuts that are *un*salted; you can eat only so much and then you will stop. Now try the salted versions. You end up consuming much more; you just cannot stop yourself from eating. The reason is very simple. The human body has a very sophisticated mechanism to tell you when to stop eating, basically like a stop sign. When you add any condiments, salt being the king of all condiments, you simply run through that stop sign. That is how you consume more food than necessary, usually empty calories along with the salt that you don't need.

In a number of studies intended to reduce high blood pressure by cutting salt in the diet, body weight also dropped along with blood pressure. This confirms what has been previously suspected, that holding off on the salt will help bring down blood pressure and unwanted pounds at the same time.

The middle-age weight gain—which we know causes all these health problems—is also not inevitable. The Yanomami

Indians are one of several tribes from the jungles of the Amazon that were not exposed to salt since birth (see INTERSALT). They remain slim and slender without automatically putting on weight in later years, as well as not having problems like high blood pressure.

You can do something about obesity and all the serious diseases that come with it.

Simply cut salt in your diet. You will cut pounds off your weight and save yourself from a great deal of misery.

Break your salt habit. You will then break the vicious cycle.

Stomach Cancer

"He passed out in the bathroom," says the wife of a seventy-year-old man brought to the ER. There are no other previous complaints. She does admit that he has not been himself for a few months—not enough energy, doesn't feel like doing things he used to enjoy doing. "There is something wrong with him. I cannot put a finger on it," she says. In the ER, a battery of tests is done; chest X-ray, CT scans of the brain, several blood tests and an EKG, etc. All of them are normal. So why did he faint?

"Wait a minute. The red blood count is too low for a man his age," says the ER doc. All expensive, sophisticated and modern tests are normal. Just a simple, old-fashioned blood test—which could have been easily overlooked—is abnormal. He is then admitted for observation and further tests. The doctors are looking for a reason for his low red blood cell count (anemia), more specifically to see if he has been losing blood slowly.

The doctors are persistent. Finally, the examination of the stomach with a scope (gastroscopy) reveals the problem. There is a large cancer in the stomach that has been bleeding slowly, causing the anemia. Unfortunately, the cancer could not be removed because it had already spread.

Cancer! That is a scary thought for anybody. Can you believe salt consumption is connected to one of the most feared cancers? Stomach cancer is the fourth leading cancer, but second leading cause of cancer deaths worldwide. It is still the number one cancer in many parts of the world including Japan, China, Korea, parts of Africa and South America. There has been no major breakthrough in the treatment of this cancer over the years. This is largely because the cancer has spread beyond cure in over 90 percent of the cases when the diagnosis is finally made.

You don't want to have any cancer, especially stomach cancer. The chances of cure are very small. While you are living with it, you can eat precious little. Eventually there comes a point when you cannot swallow even your own saliva. This is not a good way to go. Fortunately, you can cut your chances of having stomach cancer by simply cutting salt in your food.

Research has found, the more salt you add to your food, the higher the damage to the inside lining (mucosa) of the stomach. The mucosa of the stomach does not tolerate salt well at all. Once the mucosa is compromized, infection from a unique bacteria H. pylori causes stomach ulcers. As you continue to assault the stomach with salt, some of these ulcers turn into cancer. This cancer remains undiagnosed until it is too late to cure it. You are left to suffer till the eventual end.

So cut your risk of suffering one of the most miserable cancers, by simply cutting salt in your diet.

Research

Salt, salted food intake and risk of gastric cancer: epidemiologic evidence

Tsugane S. 2005. Cancer Science 96(1):1–6.

The Epidemiology and Prevention Division, National Cancer Center, Tokyo

Gastric cancer is the most common cancer in Japan. Salt intake and gastric cancer death rates are closely connected, as evaluated by 24-hour urinary sodium excretion. A validated food questionnaire also found that the higher the salt intake, the higher the incidence of stomach cancer. A similar connection between salt intake and *H. pylori* infection has also been found. *H. pylori* infection is associated with peptic ulcers.

Based on the above information, the author recommends dietary intervention with less salt consumption to prevent gastric cancer.

A prospective study of dietary salt intake and gastric cancer incidence in a defined Japanese population: The Hisayama study

Shikata K et al. 2006. International Journal of Cancer 119(1):196–201.

Kyushu University, Fukuoka, Japan

In this study, 2,476 adults were followed prospectively for 14 years. They demonstrated a significantly higher, progressively increasing incidence of gastric cancer with the amount of salt consumption. They also found strong association of high salt intake with *H. pylori* infection as well as atrophic gastritis.

Gastric cancer in Iran: epidemiology and risk factors
Malekzadeh R et al. 2009 Archives of Iranian Medicine
12(6):576–83.

Tehran University of Medical Sciences, Tehran, Iran

The authors report that gastric cancer is the most common cancer in Iran. Their research finds a strong correlation between stomach cancers in Iran and the following factors:

High intake of salt

H. pylori infection

Smoking

Gastro-esophageal reflux

For more information
about salt and other health-related issues,
please visit healthnowbooks.com.

Osteoporosis

We are at Churchill Downs, the home of the Kentucky Derby, the place to be if you are in Louisville during Derby season. A racehorse is a magnificent animal in real life, a sight to behold. The stadium comes alive all of a sudden as the race begins. Everybody is up on their feet screaming at the tops of their voices for two long minutes. I can see why people like to go to horse races, win or lose. It's exciting.

The third race of the day, the horse that came in second stumbled about 100 yards after the finish line. Very soon a large van came onto the field. The horse was put to sleep (euthanized) and carried away, right in front of me. Just like that, the rest of the day turned very sad for me. All the science and technology of the 21st century could not save a magnificent, expensive horse from a simple broken bone.

As it turns out, human beings do not fare much better after certain types of broken bones. No amount of painkillers will control the severe and persistent pain following one of these fractures. For better or worse, you cannot euthanize people like we can other animals. Unfortunately, any number of these people beg you to put them out of their misery.

Every year, more than a million Americans suffer from fractures of the bones that have become too fragile. An astounding 25 percent of the elderly die within the first year after a hip fracture. Almost all the survivors require some assistance device for mobility. Fracture of the hip most commonly affects the neck of the hip bone (see illustration). The head of the hip bone loses its blood supply and has to be replaced with an artificial joint.

Collapsed vertebrae in the spine is another very painful problem affecting more than 250,000 Americans every year. The nerves that begin in the spinal column come out though small openings on the side of the vertebra. As the vertebra collapses, the nerve is crushed. There is no easy relief from this severe pain. No wonder euthanasia comes up for discussion. You could be living in pain for the rest of your curtailed life.

In a normal bone, there is always continuous activity of building and continuous activity of breakdown. When the breakdown is going on faster than the building, the bone becomes porous, hence the name osteoporosis. Calcium is a very big part of the bone construction process. Bones affected by osteoporosis are fragile. They break very easily, even with minimal activity. Once broken, these fragile bones cannot be fixed easily, if at all.

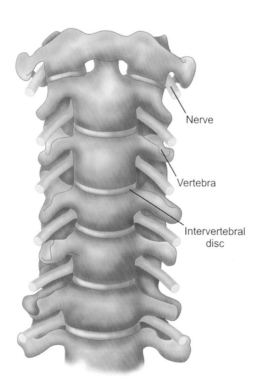

Nerve

Vertebra

Intervertebral
disc

Adding salt to your diet directly promotes osteoporosis. The human kidney cannot handle all this excess salt. In the process of trying to eliminate salt, the kidneys lose calcium in urine. The more salt you consume, the more calcium is lost by the kidneys. The construction process of the bone lags behind the breakdown process because of the decreased availability of calcium. The net result is a porous bone (see research).

Cut salt in your diet and you can reduce the risk of osteoporosis by almost a third, saving yourself from all this grief. If you have ever seen a person suffering with the pain of fractures from osteoporosis, you would never want to be in their shoes.

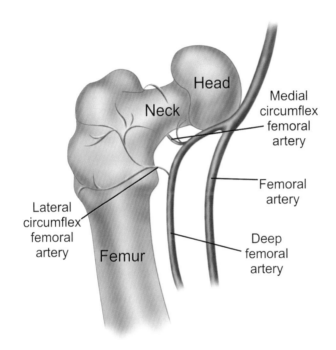

Research

The following three publications deal with salt consumption and thinning of bones, which are a significant problem in the aging population.

Thiazide effect on the mineral content of bone

Waspish RD et al. 1983. New England Journal of Medicine 309:344–347.

University of Hawaii

The mineral content of the bones was measured in 1,368 men with an average age of 68 years. Five different sites of bone were tested in each participant. Three-hundred-twenty-three men in this group were taking thiazide diuretic (water pill) for high blood pressure. This diuretic is known to reduce calcium loss in people with high blood pressure.

The mineral content of the bone was higher in the men taking thiazide diuretic than nonusers in all the five sites of bone.

Thiazide diuretics and the risk of hip fracture. Results from the Framingham Study.

Felson DT et al. 1991. Journal of the American Medical Association 265:30–373.

Boston University Arthritis Center

The authors examined the use of thiazide diuretic among 848 postmenopausal women, 176 of whom had a hip fracture. Women who were recent users of this drug were found to have a lesser incidence of hip fracture.

Low-dose hydrochlorothiazide and preservation of bone mineral density in older adults. A randomized, double-blind, placebo-controlled trial.

LaCroix AZ et al. 2000. Annals of Internal Medicine 133:516–526.

Group Health Cooperative of Puget Sound, Fred Hutchinson Cancer Research Center, and University of Washington, Seattle, Washington

The authors set up a randomized double-blind placebo-controlled study to further resolve the question of beneficial impact of thiazide diuretic on bone mineralization.

There were 320 participants followed for 3 years. At the end of this period, the treated group had a higher mineral density at both the hip and spine.

The authors conclude that the reduction of hip fractures by about one-third could be explained on the basis of thiazide diuretic use.

Memory Loss

High blood pressure can result in memory loss (dementia) in later life. Isn't that a scary thought? That is exactly what the most recent research is indicating. It is a matter of not only losing the physical functional capacities from consequences of high blood pressure; the mental functional capabilities are also affected. In the industrialized countries, disability due to mental dysfunction has become a major public health problem. Alzheimer's is the most well-known form of memory loss. Progressive loss of memory should no longer be taken as part of the normal aging process. The Alzheimer's Society is reporting a six-fold increase in memory dysfunction in people with high blood pressure; that is 600 percent higher, not just six percent!

Registration, Storage and Recall

In order to become part of the memory, a new event is first registered. This event is then stored. Recollection of this memory is the recall process. So there has to be a storage area and a communication system for proper function of the memory. Anatomically, the brain can be described as white matter (see illustration) surrounded by gray matter. The white matter is the communication system; the memory is stored in the gray matter. Damage to either part of the brain can lead to memory dysfunction.

Scans of the Brain

Routine brain scans done in people over the age of 50 have often shown small scars in both gray and white matters. The role of these fine scars is only recently becoming clear. The scars in the white matter are called white matter lesions and the scars in the gray matter are lacunar infarcts. Since a scar is an area of dead brain tissue, these marks on the brain are actually evidence of mini or silent strokes. The very small arteries at the end of the circulation system often get clogged up with cholesterol, especially in people with diabetes. High blood pressure is known to double the risk of cholesterol buildup in the arteries. This is called small vessel disease. Lacunar infarct is caused by the closure of a tiny artery. The small portion of the brain that depended upon this artery dies and is replaced by a scar. The shearing forces of high blood pressure are suspected to cause injuries to small areas of the white matter as well. These injured areas of white matter are also replaced by scars. A scar in the brain is not normal brain tissue. The scar neither stores information, nor does it communicate. Stored

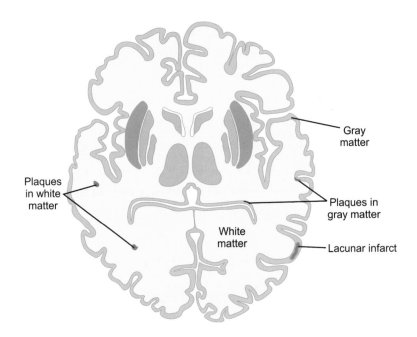

information is lost as these small scars compromise the recall process.

As researchers have found by performing periodic brain scans in people known to have these small brain scars without any symptoms (sub clinical), the development of dementia in later years is proportionate to the extent of these lesions. Not surprisingly, the extent of these lesions is also found to be proportionate to the degree of high blood pressure. Very simply, this research has shown that the higher the blood pressure, the higher the number of scars in the brain and the higher the likelihood of memory loss.

There is a certain class of high blood pressure medications known to cross the blood brain barrier, or in other words, they enter the blood circulation of the brain. These medications can do a better job of reducing blood pressure in the arteries in the brain. People who are taking these medications to control high blood pressure have been shown to have lower occurrence of memory loss in later years of life. These scientific papers are further reviewed in a later chapter. The subtle abnormalities found in routine brain scans should not be ignored anymore, just as we can no longer ignore finding enlarged heart muscle in people with high blood pressure.

Alarmed by these findings, many countries—including the United States—have launched large-scale studies. The National Institute of Health (NIH) has begun a study titled SPRINT, which is expected to enroll 7,500 people.

Research

Presence and Severity of Cerebral White Matter Lesions and Hypertension, Its Treatment, and Its Control: The ARIC Study

Duanping Liao et al 1996. Stroke 27:2262–2270.

National Institute of Health

White matter lesions (WML) and small strokes in the gray matter detected on routine scans of the brain have been reported by multiple researchers to be connected to future development of a variety of memory dysfunctions.

These authors studied the relationship between the severity of white matter lesions of the brain to the degree of high blood pressure.

The white matter lesions in 1,319 people were scored on a severity scale of 0 to 9 on MRI scans.

In the normal blood pressure group, severe lesions were noted in 7.6 percent of the scans.

In the high blood pressure group controlled by medications, severe lesions appeared in 14 percent.

In the high blood pressure uncontrolled group, severe lesions were present in 24 percent of the scans.

They also found the probability of severe WMLs increased proportionate to high blood pressure.

Use of angiotensin receptor blockers and risk of dementia in a predominantly male population: prospective cohort analysis

Nien-Chen li et al. 2010. British Medical Journal 340:b5465.

The researchers reviewed the medical records of 819,491 patients in the United States Veteran Affairs health system who were age 65 years or older and had a history of cardiovascular disease. The vast majority of participants—98 percent—were men.

From this group, over 50,000 patient records were available for study of dementia and Alzheimer's disease. They looked at progression of disease as well as mortality.

In a four-year follow-up, patients who were taking angiotensin receptor blocker (ARB) drugs were 39 percent less likely to develop dementia and 16 percent less likely to develop Alzheimer's disease, in comparison to patients taking other cardiovascular drugs. Use of another class of drugs, ACE inhibitors, was also helpful but less so compared to ARB.

Among the patients with pre-existing dementia on ARBs, nursing home admissions were lower by 39 percent and mortality lower by 11 percent.

Among the patients with Alzheimer's disease on ARBs, the risk of nursing home admission was lower by 49 percent and mortality lower by 17 percent.

Antihypertensive Treatment and Change in Blood Pressure Are Associated With the Progression of White Matter Lesion Volumes

Ophélia Godin et al. 2011. The Three-City (3C)–Dijon Magnetic Resonance Imaging Study. Circulation 123:266–273.

The authors examined the effect of high blood pressure medications on the progression of known white matter lesions. Initial MRI scans were done on 1,319 patients to document the white matter lesions. These patients were re-studied four years later by repeat MRI scan of the brain (prospective study).

In patients who had systolic blood pressure equal to or greater than 160 mm Hg, the volume of white matter lesions significantly increased to 1.60 cubic cm compared to 0.24 in patients with lower blood pressure.

Chapter

Action Plan

Now that you understand the breadth and depth of health problems you will get into when you take in too much salt, let's find out how you can go about kicking this habit.

Excuses, Excuses

I must have heard every kind of excuse since this journey began. The excuses hit the worst level when, while on an overseas trip, I was hit with a mosquito-borne virus. I had no control over the short-term illness I suffered, whereas everybody around me was indulging in self-inflicted long-term suffering from incurable diseases. What an irony!

It took me awhile to physically recover from this illness. Instead of getting upset during this time, I focused on finding ways to help salt devotees understand and follow good eating habits. As I regrouped and collected my thoughts, it occurred to me that we have to analyze these excuses comprehensively to find ways to help the reader get on the right path. So what are the impediments to getting on this path? As I methodically confront these excuses, they seem to fall into three categories.

Credibility: Why should you believe the advice I offer?

Addiction: Can you actually do it?

Action: How do you go about doing it?

Let's evaluate these questions one by one.

Credibility

There is information of all kinds out there. Much of it, however, is of questionable use and can be misleading. To get good information, like anything else in life, you have to dig deep to find it. What is so special about this book? In order to provide accurate and credible information, my son Shantanu and I pored over literally thousands of scientific publications from the last ten years. Walk into my living room, bedroom or office and you will see journals and papers everywhere. The number of hours spent on further research on the Internet is countless.

We have distilled all this complex scientific language into the chapters of this book. We have also deliberately included many scientific references to this information. A lot of our friends and early readers had a problem with these references. Understandably, this part of the book makes for boring and difficult reading. "Who is going to read this part?" our readers and editor asked us. "The reader will be turned off by this scientific gibberish and won't be able to get to the actual point." However, even after multiple revisions, we stuck to our guns.

We feel a well-informed reader is more likely to follow the

advice we offer. So we strongly encourage the reader to check out these references. The reference information can be easily copied into any Internet search engine. These efforts should make it simple for the reader to pursue further evaluation.

At the risk of sounding like I am blowing my own horn, let me also say that nobody handles more hearts than the heart surgeon. I have seen hundreds of hearts. The patient and the family know it. With each patient under our care, we go through this emotional rollercoaster ride along with the family. When things don't go right, the downhill ride is especially agonizing. We don't want you to wind up being subjected to all that we do. It is especially bothersome when we see patients return with the same problem because of their misplaced trust in pills.

Shantanu and I know that prevention is the key. This deep-rooted interest has led him to be involved in preventive care projects since his early high school days. It's what led to this book. We hope our efforts will help you to understand why you should cut salt in your food.

Addiction?

No, no, no, your salt habit is not an addiction. Smoking and narcotic use are addictions. You probably know somebody who is trying very hard to quit smoking. It's tough going. When it comes to salt, however, patches, pills, counseling, support groups, hypnotherapy, etc., are not necessary. No, you will not start shaking, get nervous, be sleepless, become cranky or simply become unable to function if you quit adding salt to your food, whether suddenly or in a slow and steady fashion. You have simply gotten used to the taste of salt. You can just as easily unlearn this habit once you set your mind to it. Those who have overcome the salt habit report enjoying their food even more. "The taste of salt masked the subtle flavors and tastes of many of my favorite foods," most people who kick their salt habit say, "I enjoy my food even more now." For taste reasons alone, those who reach this stage will protest when salt is added to their food.

Take Action

Once you get past the credibility issue and understand that it is not an addiction, you need an action plan. It is really very simple. Start slowly. Take your time. Don't give up too soon. Most people take about three months to cut salt from their diets. You will fall off the path many times. Don't get discouraged and don't compete with somebody else. Do it at your own pace.

Start with obvious sources of high salt in your daily food. Take pickles. Who needs them? You might as well eat a salt tablet. Give me a break, who cannot do without pickles? It is suicide. And what do you eat along with pickles? Yes, all those unnecessary calories. It is a double victory: less salt intake and less calorie consumption. No wonder eating less salt helps to cut the unwanted pounds you have been trying so hard to lose.

The list of common salty foods goes on.

Top Ten Most Unwanted
1. Pickles
2. Saltines and other salted crackers

3. Salted potato chips
4. Pizza made with salty dough
5. Salted nuts
6. Canned soups
7. Lunch meats
8. Many varieties of cheeses
9. Carbonated drinks
10. Boxed cereals

Boxed cereals with added salt are a pet peeve of mine. Why do you need to buy them? Many children eat cold cereal in the morning before going to school. They are not asking for salt. Why do you want to inflict long-term damage on their health? It is easy to stop this habit at an early stage.

After you've stopped using all the above salty foods, steadily cut down the amount of salt you add during food preparation. In time, you will find that you can get away with little or no salt in your food. You can do it. Many have done it.

You will reach a stage when you actually enjoy the taste of your food without salt; you don't miss or crave for the taste of salt at all. At this point, when salt is added, you actually don't like that taste anymore.

Victory!

Frequently
Asked Questions

1. *I enjoy eating. What is the point of simply living long without enjoying life? I live to eat.*

It is not only a matter of living longer; it is the quality of life in later years. As a consequence of adding salt to your food, you will have many medical, financial, and social difficulties in later years. Just about everybody will be affected, starting as early as age 50. The disabilities will be prolonged, painful, and costly. You are really not going to enjoy your later years as much as you expect to.

Secondly, most people are prescribed some dietary restriction from about the age of 50 anyway, some even earlier. They have great difficulty in adhering to such restrictions and do so begrudgingly. Transition to food with no added salt, however, is not that difficult. Once you make this successful transition, you will not miss all that excess salt. You will still enjoy the food (without salt) and be healthier as well as more functional in the long run.

2. *My tongue has grown so accustomed to the taste of salt after so many years. How can I give it up?*

The taste of salt, fortunately, is not addictive. Tobacco,

alcohol, and narcotics are addictive and not easy to forego. You may crave the taste, but there is no chemical dependency on salt. A plan of gradual decrease is likely to be successful.

3. We are already living longer and healthier lives since the industrial revolution. What is the need for this restriction?

Many anthropological studies and epidemiological studies of people across the globe, whose lifestyles are similar to that of pre-agricultural and pre-industrial populations, indicate that they do not have the same chronic illnesses as the rest of the so-called developed world. Problems of high blood pressure, diabetes, cancers, obesity, osteoporosis, etc., are uncommon in these populations. Although their average life spans are shorter, there are certainly some lessons to be learned from these studies to better our own health.

4. By how much should I reduce my salt intake?

Present data shows that even a modest reduction can be of significant benefit. The relationship between salt and blood pressure has been shown to be linear, meaning the higher the salt intake, the higher the blood pressure. Even a low level of high blood pressure over a long period of time, however, produces a lot of damage. Therefore, the best recommendation would be to get to the stage of completely eliminating added salt. Just like quitting smoking, you want to stop completely, not just cut back to ten cigarettes a day instead of twenty.

The most recent recommendation comes from the American Public Health Association (APHA), the largest association of public health professionals in the world. By a unanimous vote, the APHA passed a resolution on November 1, 2011, recommending all Americans to limit their salt intake to 1500 mg a day.

5. Isn't salt necessary for the body?

Indeed salt is necessary for the body. All the fluids of the body—including blood, sweat, and tears—are salty. But salt is already present in just about any food. There is no need to add more salt while cooking or to food already on the table.

Regulating the necessary amount of salt in the body is a task handled primarily by the kidneys. Unfortunately, our kidneys cannot get rid of all the excess salt over a prolonged period of time, which results in water retention and high blood pressure. This is the simplest way to understand how excess salt consumption causes high blood pressure.

6. Why worry about high blood pressure? Aren't there good medications these days?

There certainly are excellent medications in an ever-increasing number of categories to control high blood pressure. However, the most you can expect the medications to do is control the high blood pressure. These medications do not *cure* high blood pressure. Therefore, relying on medications is merely a false sense of security. Better to prevent high blood pressure than attempt to manage it.

There are other problems with medications:

a. The data shows that only about a third of the people who have high blood pressure are actually diagnosed, even in the developed countries. And only in about third of these people is the blood pressure adequately controlled. The odds are not great for having good control of high blood pressure in spite of advances in medicine.

b. The recommended target range to start using medications to control high blood pressure is intentionally higher than normal blood pressure—meaning you start medications for a BP reading of 140 if normal is considered 120. The normal range of blood pressure in populations who have never consumed salt is even lower (90/60). Even a low level of high BP will produce long-term damage to the heart.

c. The blood pressure control with medications does not match the natural variations and demands of the body. It may still be too high when you are resting, yet too low during activity.

d. Long-term cost of the medications has to be taken into consideration, as do possible side effects.

7. *My high blood pressure is not under control with medications. Will avoiding salt help?*

Avoiding salt has significant benefit for people with uncontrolled blood pressure and heart failure. High-salt diets contribute to high blood pressure not responding to medications. In an NIH-funded study from Australia, just one week of low-salt diet for people with resistant high blood pressure resulted in a significant reduction in blood pressure.

8. *My BP is under control with medications. Should I still avoid salt?*

Avoiding salt will help reduce the need for medications. Secondly, use of medications is not likely to regulate blood pressure in a physiological way (see above). You may have adjusted to these limitations by reducing the level of your activity, which can hurt you in the long run.

9. My blood pressure is normal and I am already 50 years old. What is the benefit of avoiding salt now?

A recent study (supported by the NIH) reported that salt reduction just for one month proportionately reduces blood pressure even in people with so-called normal blood pressure. So your normal blood pressure is actually lower than our standard levels, just as in Yanomami Indians.

10. Will risk of osteoporosis go down with avoiding salt?

Certainly. In trying to get rid of the excess salt, the kidneys lose calcium vital to bone health. A very common medication prescribed for high blood pressure, known as thiazide, has been shown to reduce calcium loss by the kidneys. Reduction in thinning of the bones at multiple body sites has been reported with thiazide use, coinciding with reduction of calcium loss. Reducing salt intake can have the same impact on osteoporosis since that will help the kidneys to retain calcium.

11. Will reducing salt intake also decrease overall food intake?

There is a natural mechanism in the body called satiety, which is responsible for telling us when we are full and don't need to eat anymore. Salt and other condiments bypass this stop sign and make you eat more. No major study is necessary on this one. Test it yourself. Try eating potato chips or peanuts with salt, and on another day try them without salt. You can eat only so many unsalted potato chips but it is difficult to stop eating the salted ones. The industry knows it—they want you to eat more and buy more. That is one reason there is so much resistance to change.

In addition, with salt and other condiments you generally end up eating so much more unhealthy food. These foods are frequently very high in empty calories with very few micronutrients. When eating only for pleasure, one should be mindful of the effect on the health of the body. In studies where body weight was also monitored, with a low salt diet, significant reduction of body weight accompanied reduction in blood pressure.

12. Is salt intake responsible for memory loss?

Yes indeed! What a shocking new finding. High blood pressure in two separate ways is responsible for small scars in the brain. Stored memory is lost and the ability to recall stored information is lost. The Alzheimer's Society is reporting a six-fold increase in dementia in people with high blood pressure.

13. I live in a hot, humid climate and I sweat a lot. Should I not compensate by adding salt to my food?

No. The kidney compensates for loss of salt from normal activity and weather by adjusting the composition of the urine. Yanomami Indians live in hot and humid Amazon jungles yet they lived for generations without adding any salt to their food. But gastrointestinal illnesses such as cholera are a different story. To replace rapid loss of fluids and salts in such illnesses, intravenous fluids of appropriate salt concentration are needed. Loss of fluids and salts during normal day-to-day activity does not require the addition of salt to the food. The kidney is fully capable of making these adjustments with the intake of only normal unsalted food.

14. Is government regulation necessary?

It is reported that nearly 80 percent or more of the excess salt consumed is already in prepackaged foods. Avoiding these foods is almost impossible for the average person. The government of Finland has reported significant improvement of cardiovascular deaths since imposing restrictions on salt in packaged foods. Other governmental agencies across the world are joining in this effort.

There is certainly much more room for the regulatory agencies to step up the protection of people from food manufacturers. For example, even if you see a bold label on the front of the box that says "0 percent fat," there is still a certain amount of saturated fat in the contents. How are you supposed to know to look for a label that says "no fat" if you don't want any fat in the package? Or you see a label that says "low salt." What the manufacturer means is that this package has lower salt than their other high-salt package. This label does not mean the salt level is truly low compared to other products that you can buy. This kind of misleading labeling is not an innocent mistake. There must be severe consequences to this type of egregious profit-first behavior in the food packaging industry to protect the average person. Confusing and misleading labeling aside, most of the excess salt in packaged foods can be regulated by various authorities.

But why depend entirely on Big Brother? Government regulation will only go so far. There is a lot you can do on your own. Don't buy a cereal that has salt added to it. The manufacturers will get the message if more and more people stop buying cereals and other food products with added salt.

Glossary

Anecdotal statement

This is a statement of personal observation, also referred to as hearsay. It is not medical proof.

Examples:

"I eat a banana every day. Therefore I don't have high blood pressure."

"I drive 70 miles an hour on this road every day and have never been stopped by a cop. So I can drive as fast as I want."

When the term "anecdotal evidence" is used, it is meant to indicate that the so-called evidence is not based on a scientific study and is therefore unreliable.

Epidemiological study

A systematic study of health problems of a given population and their eating habits is an example of this kind of study. Very valuable information is often gathered in these types of studies. For example, if a certain population has a lower blood pressure than expected and they do consume more bananas than usual, this could form a basis for further study to see if we should eat more bananas to avoid high blood pressure.

Retrospective study

Studying health problems in relation to what diet was consumed is a type of retrospective study. If the number of bananas consumed has been found to correspond to the degree of blood pressure, this information could be used to make recommendations for the future.

Prospective study

In the above example, the population was analyzed for its previous dietary habits. If this were a prospective study, the selected group would be given bananas to eat regularly and the blood pressure would be monitored.

If this type of study confirms the above findings, there will be a stronger basis for recommendation.

Prospective double-blind randomized controlled study (RCT)

This type of study is considered to provide the best evidence, the gold standard.

The study group is divided into equal groups. One group receives, for example, the medication to be tested and the other group is given a sugar pill (called a placebo).

This, of course, is hard to do this with bananas, so our example doesn't work here. In the real world, a participant does not know whether he is receiving the real thing or the placebo (blinded). The researcher who tabulates the results is also blinded, meaning he or she does not know which group is actually receiving the real medication. Results of such a study provide the highest level of evidence and form the basis for recommended treatment.

Statistically significant

When two groups are compared in a study designed as described above, the results generally are not straightforward. Not everybody in the study who eats a banana will be free of high blood pressure. Conversely, a lack of bananas in the diet will not necessarily mean that all non-banana eaters will have high blood pressure. How do you decide whether the difference in the blood pressure levels is due to the eating of bananas? These results are then subjected to statistical analysis.

Let's say 49 people in the banana group develop high blood pressure compared to 51 people in the placebo group. Could this difference be explained based on coincidence? The "p value" of this difference is determined by a statistical analysis. A high p value means there is more of a coincidental finding. As the p value decreases, the significance of the intervention increases. Scientists have generally agreed that results reach statistically significant levels starting from $p=.05$. The lower the p value, the greater the significance.

Meta-analysis

Data from several studies is analyzed by combining the data points when individual study participating numbers are small. The studies have to be dealing with the same subject matter. The findings of a meta-analysis can add more power to the conclusions of the study.

FDA approved

Manufacturers of drugs and devices make an application to the Federal Drug Administration (FDA) for approval of their use. The FDA assembles a panel of scientific experts to review the evidence presented. Only upon approval by the FDA can physicians prescribe a device or a drug. Only after this process can the manufacturer use the label "FDA Approved."

Voices in the Media

The message to cut salt has frequently surfaced in the regular news media and on the Internet, in addition to medical journals. This chapter features a small collection of the voices regularly advocating for salt reduction in the non-medical media. Reviewing this information will help reinforce the urgent need to cut excess salt consumption.

"Decrease salt in processed food and restaurant meals by 50 percent over the next 10 years."
>   —American Public Health Association, the nation's largest
>   public health organization
>   *USA Today, November 14, 2002*

"If Americans reduced their salt intake by just 1 gram per day, there would be 250,000 fewer new cases of heart disease and 200,000 fewer deaths in a decade."
>   —American Heart Association Annual Conference on Car-
>   diovascular Disease Epidemiology and Prevention 2009
>   *Carolyn Wilbert reporting for WebMD Health News,*
>   *March 11, 2009*

"End your love affair with salt; banish salt from the table and in cooking . . ."

—Dr. Simeon Margolis, John Hopkins
Posted on Yahoo Health News, June 22, 2006

"Decrease salt consumption by 50 percent over the next decade; reduce salt content in processed foods and in restaurant meals; and remove salt from the list of foods generally considered as safe so that the Food and Drug Administration could regulate the salt content of foods."
—American Medical Association
Brant McLaughlin reporting for Associated Press, November 29, 2007

"I am sure no one would tolerate so many deaths from airline crashes, so why tolerate it from food?"
—Dr. Stephen Havas, Vice President of Science and Public Health
American Medical Association
Kim Dixon reporting for Reuters, November 30, 2007

"Americans don't consume large amounts of salt because they request it, but often do so unknowingly because manufacturers and restaurants put it in . . ."
—Stephen Havas, MD, MPH, MS
American Medical Association
Brant McLaughlin reporting for Yahoo News, November 29, 2007

"There is a virtual consensus among physicians and scientists around the world that excessive sodium is one of the greatest health threats in foods. World Health Organization Forum endorses salt reduction to prevent heart disease and stroke."

> —Center for Science in the Public Interest (CSPI),
> April 9, 2007
> *www.cspinet.org*

"Clearly, salt should be considered generally recognized as dangerous, not safe."

> —Michael Jacobson, executive director, Center for Science in the Public Interest
> *Kim Dixon reporting for Reuters November 30, 2007*

"High blood pressure is a neglected disease."

> —Dr. David Fleming speaking for the Institute of Medicine and U.S. Centers for Disease Control and Prevention
> *Reported by Amanda Gardner for Healthy Day News, February 22, 2010*

"If you live long enough, you are almost guaranteed to get hypertension."

> —Dr. Corinne Huston, Institute of Medicine
> *Thomas Maugh reporting for the Los Angeles Times, February 23, 2010*

"We all consume way too much salt, and most of the salt we consume is in the food when we buy it."

> —Dr. Thomas Farley, New York City Health Commissioner
> *William Newman, New York Times, January 11, 2010*

"Salt reduction could save 92,000 U.S. lives a year: Shaving three grams off the daily salt intake of Americans could prevent up to

66,000 strokes, 99,000 heart attacks, and 92,000 deaths in the U.S., while saving $24 billion in health costs per year."

—University of San Francisco

Gene Emery reporting for Reuters Life, January 21, 2010

"The above study may underestimate the benefits [of cutting salt in our diet]."

—Dr. Lawrence Appel and Cheryl Anderson, Johns Hopkins, commenting on the above report from the University of San Francisco

Gene Emery reporting for Reuters Life, January 21, 2010

"If you don't use salt, your taste buds adjust with time . . . it took some time for one's salt-saturated taste buds to get used to low sodium level . . ."

—Joel Fuhrman, MD, June 15, 2006

www.Diseaseproof.com

"People with high blood pressure are up to six hundred percent more likely to develop dementia. One in 3 older people will end their lives with a form dementia."

—Neil Hunt, chief executive, Alzheimer's Society

Rebecca Smith reporting for The Telegraph,
September 11, 2011

"If you look . . . for things that we can prevent that lead to cognitive decline in the elderly, hypertension is at the top of the list."

—Dr. Walter Koroshetz, Deputy Director, National Institutes of Health (NIH) Institute of Neurology

Associated Press report on CNBC, January 25, 2010

The European Commission has developed an EU Framework for National Salt Initiatives. The goal of this initiative is to encourage the global population to reduce its salt intake in order to achieve the goal of World Health Organization recommendations for no more than 5 g/day. The initiative will work toward a reduction in salt of 16 percent over 4 years (4 percent per year) against the 2008 levels.

WASH

The World Action on Salt and Health (WASH) is a global entity comprised of hundreds of members from 80 countries with the mission of "improving the health of populations throughout the world by achieving a gradual reduction in salt intake." Such reductions should occur in processed foods, salt added to cooking, and salt at the table. Furthermore, one of WASH's goals is "to achieve a reduction in dietary salt intake around the world from the current intake of 10–15 g/day to the WHO target of 5 g/day." They also maintain that an "average reduction of 6 grams a day over the next decade could easily be achieved if the food industry acts." Examples of progress include New York City setting a goal of gradually reducing the amount of salt in packaged and restaurant food by 25 percent over the next five years. In the United Kingdom, the sandwich shop Subway announced that the salt levels in its products have been reduced by an average of 33 percent.

IOM

The Institute of Medicine (IOM) serves as adviser to the nation with a goal of improving health. It was established under the National Academy of Sciences and provides independent, objective, evidence-based advice to policy makers, health professionals, the private sector, and the public.

In April 2010, IOM released a report published by many news agencies entitled "Strategies to Reduce Sodium Intake in the United States" with the support of the CDC; the National Heart, Lung, and Blood Institute; the FDA; and the Department of Health & Human Services Office of Disease Prevention and Health Promotion.

The report's primary recommendation calls for the "FDA to set mandatory standards for safe levels of sodium that is added to food." Committee chairperson Dr. Jane Henney from the University of Cincinnati College of Medicine makes a plea to modify the status of salt as *generally regarded as safe* (GRAS). The report also reiterates that research has shown that salt taste preference is not only malleable, but incremental decreases in salt allows for food to be acceptable and flavorful as well. The president of the IOM, Dr. Harvey Fineberg, expressed his concern that efforts to reduce sodium intake starting decades ago have been unsuccessful.

The IOM in this report also says evidence shows that "a decrease in sodium can be accomplished successfully without affecting consumer enjoyment of food products if it is done in a stepwise process that systematically and gradually lowers sodium levels across the food supply."

"Changing consumer preferences may be the most important reason for undertaking a gradual process."

In summary, numerous prominent scientists and organizations worldwide are working hard, urging us to cut salt out of our diets.

From the behavior of the medical community and people in general, this information seems to be falling on deaf ears.

Simply telling people to quit using salt has not produced much response so far.

We hope this book will help in the fight against adding salt to our food.

For more information
about salt and other health-related issues,
please visit healthnowbooks.com.

About the Authors

Surender Reddy Neravetla, MD, FACS

Dr. Neravetla is the director of cardiac surgery at Springfield Regional Medical Center, Springfield, Ohio. This cardiac program, started by Dr. Neravetla in 1998, has received national recognition in the area of coronary artery bypass surgery for achieving the highest quality at the lowest cost. The consumer research council has recognized him as one of "America's Top Surgeons."

He graduated from Osmania Medical College, Hyderabad, India, with his medical degree. After arriving in the U.S. in 1976, he trained in general surgery at Jewish Hospital and Medical Center, Brooklyn, NY, and cardiovascular surgery at the University of Cincinnati.

Dr. Neravetla has performed nearly 10,000 cardiac, thoracic and vascular surgeries since 1983. He is known for his expertise in beating-heart surgery, valve repairs, and minimally invasive lung resections. He also has one of the largest single-surgeon experiences with one of the best results in the area of carotid surgery.

He has special interest in leading-edge robotic surgery. Dr. Neravetla is one of only a handful of surgeons who are designated as proctors for robotic lung surgery.

He has served on a number of committees inside and outside the medical field in Springfield, Ohio. The medical staff of Springfield Regional Medical Center awarded him "The Golden Stethoscope" for being the most outstanding member of the medical staff.

Shantanu Reddy Neravetla, MD

Dr. Shantanu Neravetla graduated from the University of Louisville School of Medicine. He has a Bachelor of Science with high honors from the University of Miami Honors Program. He is also a published researcher, currently doing his internship at Virginia Mason Medical Center, Seattle, Washington. Shantanu's interest in preventive health dates back to his high school years when he became one of the nation's first American Red Cross Measles Initiative National Champions to raise money and awareness for measles vaccinations around the world. In addition, he has gone on various international medical missions including serving the indigent population of Ecuador.

Coming Soon

Cut salt from your diet and you've taken a huge step toward improving your health. What is next?

- What does eating right entail?
- Why has diabetes become increasingly common, even among vegetarians?
- What is the best way to get all the vitamins your body needs?
- What are antioxidants? How do they work?
- What does the disclaimer on the bottle of your favorite vitamin supplements really mean?
- What is the single most important thing we are doing wrong with our food, other than adding salt?
- What are the only kind of carbs we should be consuming?
- Is drinking tea good for you? What is the right way and wrong way of making tea?
- Is milk good food? Is it the best way to fight osteoporosis?
- How much protection from heart disease do cholesterol-lowering pills offer?
- And finally, what kind of exercise is most beneficial?

All this and more, illustrated and explained in our next book.